20.00
-.14
E20
72548

AF778334

HIV and AIDS in the Public Schools

HIV and AIDS in the Public Schools

A Handbook for Curriculum Development, Teacher Education, and the Placement of Affected Students; With a Directory of Resources

Edited by A. ODASUO ALALI

with a foreword by B. A. Jinadu, M.D., M.P.H.

McFarland & Company, Inc., Publishers
Jefferson, North Carolina, and London

British Library Cataloguing-in-Publication data are available

Library of Congress Cataloguing-in-Publication Data

HIV and AIDS in the public schools : a handbook for curriculum
development, teacher education, and the placement of affected
students; with a directory of resources / edited by A. Odasuo Alali;
with a foreword by B.A. Jinadu.
p. cm.
Includes bibliographical references and index.
ISBN 0-7864-0135-4 (lib. bdg. : 50# alk. paper)
1. AIDS (Disease)—Study and teaching—United States—Handbooks, manuals, etc. 2. HIV (Viruses)—Study and teaching—United States—Handbooks, manuals, etc. 3. Health education—United States—Curricula—Handbooks, manuals, etc. 4. AIDS (Disease)—Patients—United States—Handbooks, manuals, etc. 5. HIV-positive persons—United States—Handbooks, manuals, etc. I. Alali, A. Odasuo, 1957–
LB3418.A35H58 1995
372.3'7—dc20 95-13439
CIP

©1995 A. Odasuo Alali. All rights reserved

Manufactured in the United States of America

McFarland & Company, Inc., Publishers
Box 611, Jefferson, North Carolina 28640

Contents

Foreword by B. A. Jinadu 1

Preface 3

Part I: Understanding the Challenge 9

1 Introduction: AIDS, Public Policy, and the Education of Students
A. Odasuo Alali 11

2 AIDS Education in the U.S. Public Schools
Hannelore Wass, M. David Miller, Gordon Thornton 20

3 Confusion Regarding HIV/AIDS and Sexual Orientation: Its Impact on the Public School System
Beth M. Rienzi, Daryl L. Hitchcock, A. Odasuo Alali 29

4 HIV/AIDS Education at a Typical Urban High School: A Teacher Survey
Fidelis Ejianreh 40

5 HIV/AIDS Education in Rural Schools
Doris Helge 51

6 HIV/AIDS Curriculum Implementation in Rural Schools: Barriers and Success
James T. Girvan, Larry D. Farrell 71

7 The Status of AIDS/HIV Education in the Professional Preparation of Preservice Elementary Teachers
David M. White, Danny J. Ballard 77

8 AIDS in the Classroom: Are Teacher Attitudes Changing?
Benjamin W. Brucker, Wayne H. Hall 85

Part II: Facing the Challenge 97

9 Placement of Students with HIV in Public Schools Policy Considerations for Educators
Wemme E. Walls 99

10 Guidelines for HIV and AIDS Student Support Services
Working Group 110

11 Integrating Community-Based Resources into AIDS Education Curricula
A. Odasuo Alali 124

12 Criteria for Evaluating AIDS Curriculum
National Coalition of Advocates for Students 130

13 Selecting and Evaluating Audiovisuals for an AIDS/HIV Education
A. Odasuo Alali 144

14 Selected Audiovisuals for HIV/AIDS Education
A. Odasuo Alali, Gary Byrd 154

15 Resources Directory for HIV/AIDS Information, Education and Prevention
A. Odasuo Alali 168

16 Suggestions for Further Reading
A. Odasuo Alali 189

About the Contributors 195

Index 199

Foreword

It was sometime in 1981 when I read the first article in the *Morbidity and Mortality Weekly Report (MMWR)* describing a skin disease, with similar characteristics, affecting four people. The article was written by Dr. Michael Gotlieb of the University of California at Los Angeles. I remember standing by the window of the cubicle of an office I was assigned as a junior faculty member of a children's hospital. I filed this article into my subconscious mind and didn't think much of it at that time other than to note briefly its epidemiologic fact and curiosity. As the issue of acquired immune deficiency syndrome (AIDS) evolved over the years and gradually caught the attention of the nation and the world, it was eerie to flash back to that afternoon with the *MMWR* in my hand and looking out that window. I have read countless articles of medical interest over the years, but I cannot recollect where I was or what I was doing, saying or wearing when I read any of the others.

Since its discovery in the early 1980s, the Human Immunodeficiency Virus (HIV), the virus that causes AIDS, has changed names; it was originally named Human T Lymphocyte Virus III (HTLV III). Our understanding of its epidemiology has changed, and it has forced society to change too, particularly in the United States. The initial epidemiological pattern seemed to be that of a disease among gay men, a group which consequently suffered a new societal backlash. That epidemiological myth was debunked when further scientific studies revealed that the mode of transmission was blood and other body fluids, thus implying that intravenous (IV) drug users were as much at risk as gay men. While society engaged in a heated morality debate about the "reason" for this disease—which by now was becoming a modern day plague—the eyes of the scientific world and the general public were suddenly opened to the fact that there were victims of the disease who contracted it through no chosen behavioral practices at all. They were the people, most especially children, who had received blood contaminated with the virus from infected donors. These secondary cases included those who received tainted blood after blood loss, particularly during surgery. There were those with blood dyscrasias such as hemophiliacs who also received contaminated blood as part of their live-saving medical treatment.

One such patient was Ryan White, the child from Kokomo, Indiana, who brought the issue of HIV and AIDS to public schools and to the attention of many who had dismissed it. The sudden and widespread public concern generated by his case (which inspired both sympathizers and persecutors) challenged politicians, public health practitioners, parents, teachers, and school administrators to design a sensible, scientifically based public policy to address this emotionally charged problem. Notwithstanding the politicization of this public health problem, and despite untold obstacles that thwart effective education to prevent the spread of HIV/AIDS, it is the education system that has, to date, been most successful in raising awareness and knowledge about the disease.

Set against this background, this book is devoted to clarifying the educational issues that AIDS raises, and to presenting strategies to help fulfill the urgent need for effective AIDS education in the public schools. The essays contained herein will be of tremendous value to educators, school administrators, public health practitioners, policy makers, and parents alike. Since that initial "public lynching" of Ryan White, schools, parents, public health officials and lawmakers have worked together continuously to create and implement effective policy. In California, for example, several pieces of legislation have allowed HIV/AIDS issues to be included in the sex education taught in schools. Senate Bill (SB) 2394 requires that wherever sex education is taught, abstinence must be emphasized. Assembly Bill (AB) 11, the AIDS prevention instruction authored by Assemblywoman Teresa Hughes and under discussion at this writing, would require school districts, county boards of education, county superintendents of schools, and the state schools for the handicapped to ensure that pupils in grades 7 through 12, or the equivalent thereof, receive AIDS prevention instruction at least once in junior high or middle school and once in high school, unless a parent or guardian requests that a pupil not attend this instruction.

This book continues that dialogue and challenges all those involved in decision or policy making to make this subject an integral part of the curriculum for future teaching professionals, particularly in elementary, middle or secondary schools. The contributors to this book are an array of professionals with a wealth of experience across many scientific and educational disciplines. They crystallize the complex issues that AIDS presents to help the reader understand and confront them.

B. A. JINADU, M.D., M.P.H.

Preface

This book tackles one of the most significant public policy issues facing American educational institutions today. The spread of AIDS has become a global problem that now affects educational institutions throughout the United States, particularly public schools. At the heart of this problem is the question of whether students infected with the human immunodeficiency virus (HIV) that causes AIDS have the legal right to attend school or to participate in school activities with students not infected with the virus. Oftentimes the resolution of this question is conditioned by what we know, do not know, or believe about people who have AIDS. Educators' responses serve as a reflection on how teachers, administrators, and parents interpret the medical information about AIDS.

Public schools now face the difficulty of balancing two equal and opposing rights: the right of a student with AIDS to an education and the right of students who are not infected with HIV to be protected against infection. The latter right is fueled by fear that one can be infected with HIV through casual contact, even though no medical evidence has found or remotely suggested that HIV can be transmitted through casual contact. The practical result of attempts to balance those rights has been to open a floodgate to discrimination against students infected with this insidious virus. Discrimination against people with AIDS must not be tolerated, because education is the best weapon we now have to fight the disease. Also, the legality of educational institutions' refusal to serve infected youths has been successfully challenged; the courts have consistently supported students' right to an education.

Schools should understand that protecting students from the adverse effects of the AIDS epidemic requires a dual strategy of prevention: educating students about the disease; and providing access or support services to those infected with HIV. This means that a school must clearly articulate its school attendance policy for children with AIDS: *all* children with AIDS must be allowed to attend regular classes; only the personal physician should act as the gatekeeper for the child's attendance at school. And the privacy of those infected with HIV should be protected, unless they choose to "go public" with their condition. There is no other acceptable perspective regarding AIDS in public schools, because the schools cannot deny students the right to an education.

Education about AIDS must start now. Educational programs should fit into the overall growth and development of children and include a successful child/ parent education format under which AIDS education is presented to parents to gain their confidence and to help them develop ways to talk to their children about AIDS. Everyone must get involved. We have no choice. Sooner or later, each of us will know someone who has AIDS or who is infected with HIV.

This book is organized in two parts. Part I, "Understanding the Challenge," contains eight chapters. It begins with an introduction, written by the editor, which analyzes HIV/AIDS in public schools within the context of policy and the student's right to education. Chapter Two examines the extent, structure, and some characteristics of education about AIDS in the U.S. public schools. The authors argue that concerted efforts in curriculum development, in-service training, and community education by schools, the medical community, and community agencies and organizations are probably most successful in bringing about effective education for school-age children. In Chapter Three, the authors examine the confusion regarding HIV/AIDS and sexual orientation, homophobia, the social fear of AIDS, physical anxiety, and their combined impact on the public school system.

Oftentimes, programmatic concerns and material selection also affect how the disease is handled in public schools. Consequently, Fidelis Ejianreh surveyed teachers at a Los Angeles high school to determine their assessment of the AIDS education and prevention programs on their campus, the reasons why they teach AIDS education, and their assessment of the materials they select for AIDS education and prevention programs. The results of this study (Chapter Four) provide the reader with insight about teachers' concerns and problems and the challenges they encounter when they teach students about AIDS and its prevention.

Chapter Five offers a balance to Ejianreh's research. Here, Doris Helge reviews some of the problems related to sexual activity among rural U.S. teenagers, successes and failures of teen sex education programs, and the problems and needs of rural areas. Helge observes that rural teens are as sexually active as their urban counterparts, yet rural areas are less likely to offer HIV education to students. Clearly, rural schools must recognize the need for effective programs to help their students delay sexual activity and to educate them about the virus that causes AIDS. Because rural schools may be limited to scarce resources, Helge suggests that they use the traditional community approach of neighbors helping neighbors, as well as cooperative extension-services. (Also see Chapter Eleven for a discussion on forging community-school relationships and Chapter Twelve on guidelines for HIV/AIDS support services.)

Along the lines suggested by Helge, James Girvan and Larry Farrell (Chapter Six) enumerate the common problems that influence the actual implementation of HIV/AIDS curricula in rural schools. They cite the following mitigating factors: fear of pressure from parents, the community, or the school administration; lack of administrative support; a failure by the community to see the AIDS crisis as "our problem"; lack of a policy that speaks to curricular issues; scarcity of state guidelines; inadequate knowledge and in-service training on how to teach about sensitive issues in the classroom; and lack of funding for materials.

Chapter Seven examines the status of AIDS/HIV education in the professional preparation of preservice elementary teachers; Chapter Eight examines the attitudes of teachers toward AIDS in the classroom. Both chapters are drawn from a survey of professional education programs and teachers.

Part II, "Facing the Challenge," is devoted to prescriptive measures to improve AIDS education in U.S. public schools, particularly as they relate to policies, selection of instructional materials, and teacher preparation. This section of the book starts with Chapter Nine, in which Wemme Walls reviews the medical and legal developments that may have implications for existing school policies. This analysis is related to the educational placement of students infected with HIV. The outgrowth of these reviews is a set of specific recommendations for decision making and policy that include awareness of pertinent state education, civil rights, and public health laws. Additionally, the chapter discusses ways that public schools can establish a vehicle for maintaining a network of resources for disseminating and utilizing new information, as well as knowledge of existing educational policies at national, state, and local levels to support educational policy and decision making. An equally important concern relates to issues of confidentiality and the infected child's right to privacy.

Chapter Ten, "Guidelines for HIV/AIDS Student Support Services," was developed by a working group representing numerous organizations. These guidelines were designed in the group's words "to encourage schools to enhance the academic and social growth of all students through the effective delivery of HIV-related student support services." The support services include school counselors, nurses, psychologists, and social workers. Although these guidelines were developed with the framework of a comprehensive support services program, they are intended also to be used in evaluating the quality of the services that schools provide. A checklist that facilitates the evaluation process is included.

Chapter Eleven argues that because of scarce resources, public schools should begin to tap the resources of the community to assist their fight against AIDS. The reader's attention is directed toward various cooperative ventures, such as community-based organizations (CBOs), and how their services can be integrated into schools' intervention programs.

This is followed by a discussion of "Criteria for Evaluating an AIDS

Curriculum" (Chapter Twelve). This chapter, written by the National Coalition of Advocates for Students, presents a set of criteria that can be used to evaluate and compare HIV curricula. It includes criteria for evaluating the developmental characteristics of students at different grade levels and appropriate approaches to HIV education in those grades. An effective staff training program and strategies for encouraging parental and community involvement are also outlined.

In Chapter Thirteen, the reader is offered a discussion of how the proliferation of media technology and the expansion of the instruments of communication have presented health educators with difficult choices concerning the appropriate means to disseminate AIDS-related information. Consequently, specific guidelines are provided for educators to use in selecting and evaluating audiovisual media for AIDS/HIV education curricula. These guidelines relate to the message objective, mode of transmission, content, visual and auditory codes, target audience, small group use, feedback capabilities, language version, ethnic and cultural appeal, and corporate author of given media.

Chapter Fourteen is a comprehensive list of selected audiovisual products for HIV/AIDS education curricula. The criteria for selecting these audiovisuals are based on those stipulated in Chapter Thirteen. As part of the effort to help educators provide accurate information about AIDS, a directory of selected resources is included as Chapter Fifteen. Public schools can use these resources to build partnerships with government and nongovernment agencies, educational and research institutions that provide HIV/AIDS information, and education and prevention services. The directory is divided into nine categories: national organizations, state public health departments, national school health programs, regional AIDS education and training centers, philanthropic organizations, expert review panels, and brochure screening consultants. Also, an extensive reading list for teacher preparation and curricula material selection is provided in Chapter Sixteen.

The job of educating America's youths has never been an easy one, and AIDS has made it even more difficult. For now, the control of HIV infection and AIDS is possible only through education that brings about behavioral change. Most public schools have not been provided with adequate resources for such school-based interventions. Therefore, more has to be done.

Our intention is not to settle this issue through this book. Additionally, this book is not intended as a forum for indictment of government institutions and leaders that have largely neglected AIDS. We hope instead to illuminate those critical issues in the age of AIDS that face America's educational system and that threaten the extinction of the human race. We hope that our work will give you, the reader, food for thought. We hope that parents of school-age children will assume a more proactive role in AIDS education and prevention. What we know, or don't know, determines how AIDS education and prevention are approached, the effectiveness of the programs that are used, and the level of risk young people face. With AIDS, students may not have a second chance to avoid infection; they deserve accurate information about the world they live in.

Writing this book was a collaborative effort. I hope that it contributes to the national debate about AIDS, and I thank and congratulate my contributors for their scholarly work.

It would have been impossible to complete this book without the help of the staff at the Centers for Disease Control, particularly Margaret Clevelan and Wilma Johnson, and Joan First at the National Coalition of Advocates for Students. In addition, I wish to express my appreciation to California Lutheran University, Thousand Oaks, for their support of this project through the Hewlett Grant.

Also, I would like to thank the following individuals for their support while I was developing the concept for this book: Dr. George Calhoun, Jr., and Dr. Bill Perry at California State University, Bakersfield; Dr. Kenoye K. Eke of Savannah State College and his wife, Joy; Francis Ero and Wilson Gambe of Bakersfield, California; Dr. Beverly Kelley and Professor Loran Lewis at California Lutheran University; B. A. Jinadu, M.D., M.P.H., Health Officer and Director of Public Health for the County of Kern, California; K. Reuben Uku, M.D., of Kaiser Permanente, Los Angeles; Charles Ibrahim of GTE Corporation; Dr. Nicholas A. Okpekho at University of New Mexico and Mr. Eric Abi and Jeffry K. Eke of Atlanta, Georgia. I am grateful to Chris Kelly for reading the first draft of some of the chapters in this book. His suggestions are appreciated.

I must also acknowledge the love and support of my parents, Unice and Andrew; my brothers, Harcourt, Kenoye, Akari, Umor, and Idiowa and my sisters, Enighe, Ilami, Daima, and Ikpoki (and her husband Clinton).

This book is dedicated to the Ryan Whites who never gave up the fight to preserve the educational rights of students with AIDS. Your struggles shall never be forgotten.

A. Odasuo Alali

Part I
Understanding the Challenge

Chapter One

Introduction: AIDS, Public Policy, and the Education of Students

A. ODASUO ALALI

The AIDS epidemic, now well into its second decade, has relentlessly expanded in scope and magnitude since 1981, when the disease was first diagnosed. In that first year there were 298 cases reported by the Centers for Disease Control (CDC). By the end of 1990, however, the nation's disease prevention agency reported 43,339 cases of the disease for that year (Noble, Parran, & Holman, 1991); the number of AIDS cases in 1994 was 80,691 (CDC, 1994). The CDC (1990a, p. 117) estimates that between 1 million and 1.5 million Americans carry the human immunodeficiency virus (HIV or HIV-1) that causes AIDS. Projections from extensive HIV seroprevalence studies suggest that the HIV infection rate will probably double, if not quadruple, by the year 2000.

Acquired immunodeficiency syndrome, which results from infection with HIV, has now become one of the leading causes of death in the United States. Between 1981 and 1994, the number of persons who died of AIDS multiplied several thousand times: The CDC documented only 164 AIDS-related deaths in 1981; by the end of 1994, the disease had claimed a cumulative total of 270,870 lives. The World Health Organization reported that AIDS cases worldwide increased from 2.5 million to 4 million in just 1993; in the U.S. for the same year, there were 106,618 AIDS cases (CDC, 1994, p. 5). These figures paint a dismal picture.

One of the primary risk groups for HIV infection is teenagers. Two CDC surveillance reports (1990b, p. 12; 1989, p. 11) show that between January 31, 1989, and February 1, 1990, the number of cases among 13- to 19-year-olds increased by 40 percent. Additionally, 20 percent of the AIDS patients have been between the ages of 20 and 29 (CDC, 1990c, p. 12), and AIDS is now the sixth leading cause of death among those 15 to 24 years of age. The AIDS cases continue to increase: in 1994 alone, the CDC reported 82 percent of AIDS cases were among male adults/adolescents (1994, p. 5). Because the incubation period for the virus is 10 years or more, it is reasonable to suppose that a majority of these persons were infected during their teenage years. Perhaps the most troubling aspect is that because teenagers feel invulnerable, they often exhibit risky behavior (unprotected sex, use of illegal drugs, alcohol abuse, and prostitution) that increases their chance of infection with HIV.

In a preliminary study of 285 Baltimore inner-city teenage girls 12 to 18 years old, 9 out of 10 said they knew that unprotected sex put them at risk for AIDS, yet only 4 in 10 said they had asked their partners to use condoms the last time they had intercourse ("Preliminary Study," 1988, p. 7). Three weeks after Earvin "Magic" Johnson revealed that he had tested positive for HIV, Who's Who Among High School Students conducted a nationwide "AIDS Survey of High Achievers" (Husted & Kennedy, 1992, p. 13). The results of this survey show that only 22 percent of the 1,150 A- and B-average students surveyed were either "worried" or "very worried" about contracting HIV. Nearly half of the sexually active students (42 percent) said they would have intercourse even if they or their partner did not have a condom. It is no wonder that 1 in 100 teens in Miami and New York has the AIDS virus; in rural areas, the infection rate is 0.3 per 100 ("Schools Can Help," 1990, p. A-12). More evidence of the impact of teenage sexual behavior is provided in a study published in the *New England Journal of Medicine* (Quinn et al., 1988). The study shows that 2.5 percent of the 434 females and 2 percent of the 509 males (15 to 19 years old) who visited Baltimore clinics for treatment of sexually transmitted diseases (STDs) were infected with HIV-1.

Clearly, teenagers are a critical group for infection with HIV, and convincing them to modify their behavior is a public health educator's challenge. "We are facing a critical public health challenge in the 1990s" (CDC, 1990d), says Dr. William L. Roper, director of CDC. This challenge is compounded by the lack of medical breakthroughs in prevention of the disease. With the increasing rate of teenage infection, HIV and AIDS now present some of the most significant public policy issues facing the American educational system: how to treat students and personnel with the virus; the primary goals of AIDS education; what prevention measures to suggest to students (e.g., abstinence, safe sex, or both); teacher preparation and material selection; and whether a given AIDS curriculum is culturally sensitive.

How to Treat Students and Personnel with HIV

Harney (1990, p. 827) observes that "no single issue better frames the central concerns of public policy as it relates to the treatment of persons with AIDS than the controversy over the presence in public schools of students who are infected with the AIDS virus." Because this concern has created hysteria, AIDS in public schools has been placed on the national agenda. As in most controversial issues, the hysteria over students with AIDS is often replayed in the media whenever the former are denied access to education in U.S. public schools.

Of the cases that have been replayed in the media, the one that received the most extensive coverage was that of Ryan White, a Kokomo, Indiana, teenager who died in 1990 (Harney, 1990, p. 828). Although the Ryan White news stories catapulted this issue to national prominence, there were legal arguments in courts that provided some relief to students with AIDS. In a New York case, a local school board sought to enjoin a New York City Board of Education decision to allow an anonymous 7-year-old child with AIDS into a public school classroom in the borough of Queens. The decision provoked a lawsuit against the board of education (*District 27 Community School Board v. Board of Education*). The trial court ruled in favor of the board of education, asserting that "there is no factual basis or legal basis for excluding children with AIDS from school" (Schwarz & Schaffer, 1985, p. 173). Though court decisions have not resolved the issue at the local school level, administrators must realize that they are legally bound to provide students and personnel who are infected with HIV equal access to medical and social services, employment, housing and educational opportunities.

Students who are refused these services may seek refuge under Section 504 of the Rehabilitation Act of 1973, which entitles handicapped persons to education in schools:

> No otherwise qualified handicapped individual in the United States ... shall, solely by reason of his handicap, be excluded from participation in, be denied the benefits of, or be subjected to discrimination under any program or activity receiving Federal financial assistance [29 U.S.C. Sec. 794].

Although the Supreme Court decision in *School Board of Nassau County v. Arline* concluded that a person with a contagious disease is handicapped under Section 504, a few school districts have sought to challenge the provisions of the section. Most of them have failed. In *Ray v. School District of DeSoto County*, a judge ordered the school district to enroll three brothers, all hemophiliacs with the AIDS virus, in a regular classroom setting "unless and until it could be established these children posed a real and valid threat to the school population of DeSoto County." A California court also blocked a legal maneuver to remove Ryan Thomas, a kindergarten student with HIV, from his class after he bit another child during an altercation (*Thomas v. Atascadero Unified School District*).

Clearly, the question as to whether students and personnel with HIV infection have equal access or rights to educational opportunities should be considered moot. There is no legal basis for excluding them from school activities. Wemme Walls sheds more light on this perspective in Chapter Nine.

The Primary Goals of AIDS Education

Another policy issue that confronts the public school system pertains to the confusion regarding the educational objectives of AIDS prevention programs. Clearly, AIDS education at all grade levels should be the cornerstone of any prevention program. The scope and content of AIDS education should be determined by the dialogue that takes place between the school and its community, including parental concerns. There is no obvious reason for disconnection between a school and its community, especially with AIDS. A prevention program should also encompass a comprehensive sexuality education that emphasizes sexual knowledge, beliefs, attitudes, values, and behaviors of individuals. It should also include discussions about decision making and communication. More important, it must be culturally sensitive and utilize the linguistic codes that are recognized by the target population (see the section in this chapter on "Culture and AIDS in the Curriculum," p. 17). In short, what happens in the classroom, the organization and structure of the classroom, and instructional or educational issues and objectives should be shaped by these interactions and other mitigating variables.

Most schools already recognize that they must play a pivotal role in AIDS prevention. A survey by the National School Boards Association shows that as of 1990 almost 80 percent of the nation's public schools already provided HIV/AIDS education and prevention programs ("Survey Shows," 1990, p. 5). Of the 332 school districts that were surveyed for this study, 20 percent said they started AIDS prevention instruction during the 1986-87 school year, 32 percent in 1987-88 and 37 percent in 1988-89. Also, 85 percent said they required HIV education for seventh graders, and 58 percent for twelfth graders. As of March 1992, only 17 states mandated and 30 states recommended sexuality education, but 34 states mandated and 14 recommended HIV/AIDS education (Haffner, 1992, p. 3).

Although a majority of the public schools have school-based programs, they must realize that the fundamental objective of their AIDS education is to impact knowledge and thereby change behavior—in other words, the goal is prevention. Numerous organizations, including the Center for Population Options (Haffner, 1987, p. 3), have suggested specific goals for AIDS education:

- to reduce the panic and misinformation about the disease and its transmission;
- to help teenagers delay the initiation of sexual intercourse;
- to ensure that teenagers who are having any type of intercourse use condoms consistently and effectively; and
- to reduce experimentation with drugs and prevent IV drug use.

Additionally, because AIDS is a stigmatized disease, it is incumbent upon schools to provide their students with correct data and support services that will help to dispel the myths and to reduce anxiety and fears associated with the disease.

Perhaps the best way to determine the effectiveness of any AIDS education program is to review it periodically. Diane de Mauro (1989-1990, p. 5), the director of program services at the Sex Information and Education Council of the United States (SIECUS), suggests the following elements that educators can look for in reviewing their AIDS education curricula:

- an assessment of the accuracy of information provided;
- coverage of abstinence and safer sex as preventive practices;
- description of condom use;
- discussion of homosexuality, as governed by a specific definition;
- emphasis on risk behavior versus risk groups;
- presentation of sexuality as a natural part of human life; and
- presentation of the variety and range of human sexual behavior.

Additional guidelines for HIV and AIDS student support services in schools are provided in Chapter Ten.

Preventive Measures

The question foremost on the minds of students concerned with HIV infection is, "What can I do to keep from contracting HIV?" Out of this question comes a dilemma for some educators: what preventive measures to suggest for their students. This is because the debate that is associated with AIDS education and prevention often devolves into what is or is not "politically correct." Few preventive measures that teachers might suggest are simultaneously acceptable to parents, the religious-right watchdogs, the conservative leadership that believes AIDS education may promote promiscuity among teenagers, and more liberal groups. The question therefore is whether educators should prescribe abstinence, safe sex, or both.

It is unrealistic only to suggest abstinence, because students are engaging in sexual activities at early ages. It is more realistic, however, for teachers to suggest the following four preventive measures for their students (National Coalition of Advocates for Students, 1990, p. 41): abstain from sexual intercourse, practice sexual fidelity with an uninfected partner, use latex condoms and a spermicide when engaged in sexual intercourse, and do not use intravenous drugs or share needles or syringes.

Teacher Preparation and Material Selection

The fourth issue that confronts schools pertains to the professional preparation—or the lack of it—of those who teach AIDS and sex education. This is a legitimate educational concern, because the degree to which teachers are trained or prepared to teach students about the disease may have a tremendous impact on the materials they select and on how messages are prepared and communicated. In their analysis of what public school teachers teach about preventing pregnancy, AIDS, and STDs, Forrest and Silverman (1989) found that because sex education teachers lack appropriate teaching materials, they tend to develop their own teaching materials and, in the process, to increase the danger of disseminating inaccurate information about AIDS. Although no study has yet determined the prevalence of this phenomenon, such actions could nurture an environment for confusion and fear of the disease or those who have it.

There is also no doubt that teacher preparation is pivotal to AIDS education, and that this affects the materials teachers select for AIDS education. The issue then becomes how best to prepare teachers to educate their students about AIDS. Though most teachers believe that formal training may not be necessary for those who teach AIDS education (see Chapter Four), teacher preparation is necessary to ensure that accurate information is disseminated. This type of preparation can take many forms:

1. Basic teacher training programs and seminars that are designed to prepare teachers to teach students about HIV and AIDS. These trainings could be in the form of in-service courses, continuing education courses, or short-term seminars (Moglia, 1989-1990).
2. Advanced teacher training in the form of academic courses or programs that lead to a specialization in teaching AIDS and human sexuality.
3. Informal education wherein teachers familiarize themselves with the state and school system policy on HIV/AIDS education and new developments in the area.
4. Collaborating with self-help organizations that would provide additional teaching materials (brochures, films, pamphlets, etc.) and student services that include counseling and community outreach programs.
5. Familiarization with parental concerns that discussions about HIV or AIDS may encourage their children to initiate sexual activity at an early age. All teachers should also acquaint themselves with the school's parental notification policy and devise ways to involve parents in AIDS education. (See accompanying sample letter to parents.)
6. Fostering a comfortable and trusting classroom atmosphere in which controversial and sensitive AIDS-related issues can be discussed.

Sample Letter to Parents

Dear Parent or Guardian:

AIDS is a very serious health problem. Young people can get it through sex or using drugs. Beginning ______________, your
(date)
child will be taking a health class on AIDS.

You are invited to a meeting for parents. It will be held on
__________________ at ______________ at ____________.
(time) (place)
At this meeting, we will talk about AIDS and what your child will be learning at school. We will show you the lessons that will be taught. You can ask any questions that you have.

You can help at home by talking with your child about how to prevent AIDS. This meeting can help you learn to do that.

We hope that you can come.

Sincerely,

____
(Principal)

____
(Teacher)

Reprinted with permission from National Coalition of Advocates for Students, Boston, Massachusetts.

It is also important for the local school board and trustees to create an environment that will foster creative development of their teachers. A comprehensive approach is required in preparation for AIDS education.

Culture and AIDS in the Curriculum

Culture plays a pivotal role that determines the effectiveness of AIDS education and prevention programs. As Worth (1990) observes, "Culturally determined values influence how individual perceptions of AIDS are selected, how attitudes toward high-risk behavior are formed, how habits that characterize high-risk behavior are developed, and how risk-reduction information will be processed" (p. 111). Clearly, to dislodge cultural values from AIDS education and prevention is to ignore "the medium through which sexuality, drug use, and disease are interpreted and acted upon" (p. 111).

As public schools are confronted with this issue, they must strive for cultural sensitivity by recognizing that the American society is made up of diverse cultural groups. There is no dominant set of cultural values. Campaigns for AIDS education would be easier if we belonged to only one culture, but because this is not the case, no catch-all AIDS curriculum can suffice. Schools that do not recognize this fact run the risk of excluding ethnic groups such as Latinos and African-Americans in their AIDS education programs.

In other cases where cultural values of a diverse student body are not considered in AIDS education, the messages may be offensive to a specific ethnic group. In one case, an educational campaign that was originally offensive to African-Americans was redesigned to include their viewpoints (Herscher, 1991). Culture and AIDS are inseparably linked. Therefore, a school AIDS curriculum should be sensitive to the ethnically diverse student population it serves.

Once these concerns are adequately resolved, teachers will find it much easier, barring budgetary problems, to go about providing quality AIDS education for their students. It is also my strong contention that these issues will not be resolved adequately if schools do not reconcile their educational objectives with the prevailing attitudes of the immediate communities where their schools are located and with the attitudes of teachers, administrators, and the local school board of trustees. In the end, they shape how the community reacts, what goes on in the classroom, and how students are educated about the disease.

In order to tackle these and other significant public policy issues that face the American educational system today, we rely on the contributions of distinguished scholars and organizations. Through these articles, we hope to reflect these issues adequately so as to bridge the gap that now exists between educational choices, what is delivered to students, and the treatment of students with HIV. We attempt not only to examine specific policies on HIV and AIDS in public schools, but to provide the reader with analyses of policies within the context of students' right to education. Implicit here is the need to fill the void that currently exists between public policy, curriculum guidelines, and curriculum implementation. Explicit are the implications for researchers, educators, policy makers, and curriculum planners.

References

Centers for Disease Control (1989, February). *HIV/AIDS Surveillance.*

____ (1990a). "Estimates of HIV Prevalence and Projected AIDS Cases: Summary of a Workshop, October 31–November 1, 1989." *Morbidity and Mortality Weekly Report,* 39.

____ (1990b, February). *HIV/AIDS Surveillance Report.*

____ (1990c, March). *HIV/AIDS Surveillance Report.*

____ (1990d). *CDC HIV/AIDS Prevention Factbook.* Atlanta, GA: CDC.

Centers for Disease Control (1994). *HIV/AIDS Surveillance Report,* 6:2; (1–39).

de Mauro, D. (1989-1990, December-January). "Sexuality Education 1990: A Review of State Sexuality and AIDS Education Curricula." *SIECUS Report,* 18(2):1–9.

District 27 Community School Board v. Board of Education, 130 Misc. 2d 398, 502 N.Y. 2d 325 (Sup. Ct. 1986).

Forrest, J. D., and Silverman, J. (1989). "What Public School Teachers Teach About Preventing Pregnancy, AIDS and Sexually Transmitted Diseases." *Family Planning Perspectives,* 21(2):65–72.

Haffner, D. W. (1992, February-March). "1992 Report Card on the States: Sexual Rights in America." *SIECUS Report,* 20(3):1–7.

____ (1987, November). *AIDS and Adolescents: The Time for Prevention Is Now.* Washington, DC: Center for Population Options.

Harney, D. M. (1990, December). "Legal Advocacy as a Means of Defining Social Policy: Arguing School Admissions for Children with AIDS." *Communication Research,* 17(6):827–841.

Herscher, J. (1991, March 2). "New AIDS Information Campaign." *San Francisco Chronicle,* Sect. A24.

Husted, A., and Kennedy, S. (1992, February 18). "Students Do Poorly in High School AIDS Survey." *Atlanta Journal/Constitution,* p. 13.

Moglia, R. (1989-1990, December-January). "The Professional Preparation of Sexuality Educators: A Pivotal Factor for Sexuality Education." *SIECUS Report,* pp. 13–15.

National Coalition of Advocates for Students (1990, May). *On the Road to Healthy Living: A Bilingual Curriculum on AIDS and HIV Prevention for Migrant Students (Grades 6–12).* Boston, MA: NCAS.

Noble, G. R.; Parra, W. C.; and Holman, P. B. (1991, November-December). "Organizational Structure and Resources of CDC's HIV-AIDS Prevention Program." *Public Health Reports,* 106(6):604–607.

"Preliminary Study Results Suggest Teenage Girls Engage in High Risk Sex in Spite of Knowledge of AIDS" (1988, November 15). *AIDS/HIV Record,* 2(9).

Quinn, T. C.; Glasser, D.; Cannon, R. O.; Matuszak, D. L.; Dunning, R. W.; Kline, R. L.; Campbell, C. H.; Israel, E.; Fauci, A. S.; and Hook, E. W., III (1988, January 28). "Human Immunodeficiency Virus Infection Among Patients Attending Clinics for Sexually Transmitted Diseases." *New England Journal of Medicine,* 318(4):198–203.

Ray v. School District of DeSoto County, 666 F. Supp. 1524 [4 Ed. Law Rep. 632] (M.D. Fla. 1987).

School Board of Nassau County v. Arline, 107 S.Ct. 1123 (1987).

"Schools Can Help Teens Deal with Sex" (1990, May 17). *USA Today* (editorial), p. 12A.

Schwarz, F. A., and Schaffer, F. P. (1985). "AIDS in the Classroom (Law, Social Policy, and Contagious Disease: A Symposium on Acquired Immune Deficiency Syndrome)." *Hofstra Law Review,* 14:163–191.

"Survey Shows Four of Five Public Schools Teach HIV Prevention" (1990, April 30). *AIDS/HIV Record,* 4(1):5.

Thomas v. Atascadero Unified School District, 662 F. Supp. 376 [40 Ed. Law Rep. 732] (C.D. Cal. 1986).

World Health Organization (1987). *Special Program on AIDS: Strategies and Structure Projected Needs.* Geneva: WHO.

Worth, D. (1990). "Minority Women and AIDS: Culture, Race and Gender." In D. A. Feldman, ed., *Culture and AIDS,* p. 111–135. New York: Praeger.

Chapter Two

AIDS Education in the U.S. Public Schools

HANNELORE WASS
M. DAVID MILLER
GORDON THORNTON

Educators have long advocated sex education in the public schools although surveys indicate that only a small proportion of the schools have actually provided it (Kirby, Alter, & Scales, 1979; Kirby, 1980), despite favorable attitudes on the part of parents (Yarber, 1979) and the public in general (Gallup, 1981; Louis Harris & Associates, 1988). With the discovery and spread of AIDS, the issue has taken on a dramatic urgency. It is estimated that thousands of teenagers are at risk of contracting the human immunodeficiency virus (HIV) that causes AIDS because they engage in risky sexual behavior or drug use, or both (American School Health Association et al., 1988). Currently one-fifth of the people with AIDS are in their twenties (United States Department of Education, 1988; American School Health Association et al., 1988), many of them perhaps having contracted the disease during adolescence.

Adolescents, while aware of the risks of AIDS, have important misconceptions about this disease (American School Health Association et al., 1988). Former Surgeon General C. Everett Koop in his *Surgeon General's Report on AIDS* (1986) and his address to the California Legislature (1989) advised strongly that AIDS education be part of the public schools' regular curriculum and that it begin at the elementary school level. The Presidential Commission on the Human Immunodeficiency Virus Epidemic made the same recommendation in its report (1988). Furthermore, the Committee on School Health of the American Academy of Pediatrics (1988), the Coalition of National Health Education Organizations (1988), the American Association of School Adminis-

This article was originally published in AIDS Education and Prevention, *2(3), pp. 213–219 (1990). Reprinted by permission of Guilford Press.*

trators (Keough, 1988), and the Citizens Commission for AIDS for New York City and Northern New Jersey (1989) recommended that schools provide instruction about AIDS as part of a comprehensive health education program for kindergarten through grade 12. Thus major responsibility for AIDS education appears to be delegated to health educators. The U.S. Department of Health and Human Services, in collaboration with the Public Health Service, the Centers for Disease Control, and the Center for Health Promotion and Education (1988), has developed comprehensive guidelines for school health education programs at all levels to prevent the spread of AIDS. Schools across the country are apparently developing AIDS education programs (Lansford, 1988). And the number of state departments of education that require AIDS education has been increasing rapidly. In a state-by-state survey conducted by the National Association of State Boards of Education (Fraser & Mitchell, 1988) it was found that 23 states and the District of Columbia mandate AIDS instruction. According to a survey conducted by the Alan Guttmacher Institute, 31 state departments of education require instruction about AIDS (Kenney, Guardado & Brown, 1989). Others are highly active in promoting such instruction even though they do not mandate it. States that mandate AIDS instruction vary, however, in their approach to the execution of this instruction. While most states mandate AIDS instruction as part of their comprehensive health education program, a few require that it be part of sex education, instruction on a sexually transmitted disease or a communicable disease, or by itself (Fraser & Mitchell, 1988).

Yet there are very few studies that have investigated what is actually done by way of AIDS education in our nation's public schools. Recently the Alan Guttmacher Institute conducted a survey of sex education including education about preventing pregnancy, AIDS, and sexually transmitted disease at the high school level in large urban districts. The researchers found that 77 percent of the schools offer sex education and AIDS education and that such education tends not to occur until the ninth or tenth grade (Forrest & Silverman, 1989). Because of their focus on large school districts, in grades 7 to 12, a national estimate of AIDS education across all grade levels and school sizes was not available. The purpose of the present study was to conduct such a survey to determine the extent, structure, and some characteristics of education about AIDS in the U.S. public schools. The survey was conducted during the 1987-88 school year.

Method

Sampling A stratified (by region) random sample of 1,000 schools, prekindergarten/kindergarten through grade 12, from 1986-87 U.S. Department of Education list of 81,049 regular elementary and secondary schools were mailed

Figure 2.1: AIDS Education Questionnaire

1. Are you a
   a). teacher? __ b). school counselor? __ c). other? __
   Please identify your position. ______________________

2. Does your school have an AIDS education program? Yes __ No __
   If No, please skip to Question 9.

3. List all grade levels at which this program is taught. ______________

4. Is the program offered in the entire school district? Yes __ No __

5. Who directs the program?
   a). health educator __
   b). a physical education teacher __
   c). a team of school staff __ (Please list positions.) ______________
   d). an outside expert __ (Please identify.) ______________
   e). other __ (Please identify.) ______________

6. Which of the following are components of the program? (Please check all that apply.)
   a). ways of transmittal of AIDS __ d). mortality __
   b). prevention __ e). fears of contracting AIDS __
   c). treatment __ f). other __
   (Please describe.) ______________

7. What curriculum materials do you use? Please check all that apply:
   a). published printed material __ (Please give author, title, and publisher.)
   ______________________ *
   b). material developed by school staff ______________ *
   c). material developed by school staff and medical professionals __
   d). other __ (Please explain.) ______________ *

8. Do the parents support this program? Yes __ No __

9. Please share any experiences and thoughts you have on AIDS education. *

If you want a summary of this survey, please print your name and address below: ______________________

____

____

If you or your colleagues have developed your own curriculum materials, we would appreciate receiving a copy. Thank you!

*Note: Additional space was provided on original questionnaire.

---

a questionnaire. A second mailout was made to a random sample of 500 of the non-responding schools. A cover letter to the principals requested that the questionnaire be given to the appropriate school personnel to answer. Two hundred twenty-two schools responded to the mailouts. A random sample of 217 non-responding schools was then selected for telephone interviews. Of these, 16 schools either could not be contacted (n=8) or refused (n=8). The telephone interviewer, one of the authors, read the questions as they appeared on the questionnaire and recorded the responses accordingly. The mailed response rate was fairly low (22.2 percent). However, that of the telephone survey was 93 percent. The respondents in the survey were similar to the population by region. Table 1 shows that the sample had a small over-representation from the Midwest (36 percent vs. 31 percent) with a corresponding under-representation from the East and West combined. The respondents were also similar to the population by grade level in the school.

Table 2.1: Stratified Sampling Design

Region	*Population %**	*Sample*	*Return n*	*Return %*
East	18.5	185	67	16.3
Midwest	30.6	306	150	36.4
South	21.4	214	88	21.3
West	29.5	295	107	26.0

*This is drawn from the U.S. Department of Education list of public elementary and secondary schools.

Instrumentation An AIDS education questionnaire was developed by the authors of this study. The questionnaire was reviewed by health professionals and educators. The final instrument is reproduced in Figure 2.1.

Analyses Consistently fewer schools in the telephone survey sample reported having AIDS education programs than did schools in the mail-in sample, suggesting that schools that did not respond to the mailings are less likely to have AIDS education programs than are those that responded. With the low return rate in the mail-in sample (22.2 percent) and the high return rate in the phone sample (93 percent), the phone sample was treated as an unbiased estimate of the percent of programs in the sample that did not mail in. Thus, the national estimate for AIDS education was the following weighted composite of the two samples:

$$\frac{222\ \{\%\text{ AIDS Program (Mail)}\} + 778\ \{\%\text{AIDS Program (Phone)}\}}{1000}$$

Because of the higher weight for the phone sample, where the percent of AIDS programs is lower, the national estimate was lower than the total sample percent.

Descriptive statistics were reported for prevalence of AIDS education by region and grade level. Finally, percentages were reported for the follow-up questions to describe the AIDS education programs.

Results

As expected, the prevalence of AIDS education was higher in the initial mail-in sample (52.70 percent) than in the phone sample (43.78 percent). The weighted national estimate for AIDS education was 45.76 percent. In the sample, 205 schools reported having an AIDS education program. The distribution of these schools by geographic region is presented in Table 2.2. The largest percentage of AIDS programs in offered in the East and the smallest in the South. The distribution of AIDS programs by "highest grade" is shown in Table 2.3. "Highest grade" refers to the highest grade included in a particular school. For example, all schools in which the highest grade is 7, 8, or 9 are listed in the "highest grade" category 7–9 regardless of the lower grades that may or may not be offered in that school. A school with grades 4–8 would be included in the 7–9 category. The largest percentage of AIDS programs is offered in grade levels 10–12. The percentages at the other grade levels are similar to each other. Nearly all the schools that have AIDS education report that their programs are offered in the entire school district.

Table 2.2: Distribution of AIDS Education Programs by Geographic Region*

	Schools	
Region	*n*	%
East	44	65.7
Midwest	76	50.7
South	33	37.5
West	45	42.1

*Some respondents did not provide this information.

In follow-up questions to show the characteristics of existing AIDS education programs, there were no statistically significant differences between the mail-in and the phone samples. Thus, the results of these questions are unweighted composites of the two samples.

Almost half of the respondents said that their program is taught by a health educator (46.4 percent), about a fourth by a team of school staff (24.7 percent), and a few by physical education teachers (4.2 percent), an outside expert (3.6 percent) or other personnel such as the nurse, curriculum director, or AIDS

Table 2.3: Distribution of AIDS Education Programs by "Highest Grade" Level

	Schools	
Highest Grade	*n*	*%*
10–12	72	61.0
7–9	49	47.1
PK–6	77	40.5

*Some respondents did not provide this information.

advisory council. Twenty-two of the schools reported the composition of the team involved in AIDS education. The most frequently mentioned team members were teachers, followed by counselors and nurses and lastly administrators.

Components of the programs in rank order were prevention (81 percent), transmittal (79 percent), fears of contracting AIDS (65 percent), mortality (56 percent), and treatment (53 percent). Other components listed by some schools were abstinence and myths about AIDS. Forty-six percent of the respondents reported using published materials, 38 percent materials constructed by school staff, and 30 percent material constructed jointly by school staff and medical professionals. Other materials used (18 percent) were curriculum guides developed by the state and various audiovisuals. Nearly all respondents (97 percent) said that parents support their programs. As an illustration of this support a number of schools reported that parents could have their child excused from the AIDS classes but rarely exercise this option.

Discussion

Our results indicate that nearly half of the nation's public schools provide some form of education about AIDS. Given its lethality and rapid spread, the vulnerability of our youth, and the straightforward, vigorous leadership of former U.S. Surgeon General Koop (1986, 1989), this is not surprising. While Forrest and Silverman (1989) reported higher levels of AIDS education, their study was limited to the largest school districts in grades 7–12. Our study suggests that AIDS education is less prevalent in lower grade levels and smaller schools. Continuing efforts by government officials, health professionals, and school personnel are needed to convince all educators that such education is necessary.

As Koop noted (1986), before we can educate our children about AIDS we must educate ourselves. Notably, 16 million copies of Everett Koop's *Surgeon General's Report on AIDS* and 107 million copies of an AIDS pamphlet (U.S. Department of Health and Human Services, 1988) are in print with the effects of the latter currently being evaluated (Centers for Disease Control, 1989). The need for knowledge is also apparent from a recent survey of health educators (Kerr, Allensworth, Gayle & Dalis, 1989). Sixty percent of the respondents said they needed information on how to promote or plan AIDS education programs. Nearly half needed help in evaluating resource materials. A number of respondents showed knowledge gaps concerning AIDS, although they scored higher than the general public. Teachers apparently recognized this lack: Nearly two-thirds of the respondents in the above survey said that they needed in-service education. In their survey Forrest and Silverman (1989) found that 65 percent of the teachers who provide instruction on AIDS need instructional materials. In this connection, it should be noted also that while many state education agencies have given clear mandates for AIDS instruction, state funding for training and other assistance to local schools has been lacking (Fraser & Mitchell, 1988).

Although health officials (e.g. Koop, 1986, 1989) and professionals (e.g. American Academy of Pediatrics, 1988; Coalition of National Health Education Organizations, 1988) have urged developmentally appropriate AIDS instruction for the lower grade levels beginning with kindergarten, a number of state departments of education do not mandate it until high school (Fraser & Mitchell, 1988; Kenney et al., 1989), and school superintendents disagree on the educational levels at which it should occur (Ficklen, 1988). Our data seem to reflect this disagreement showing that substantially fewer schools provide AIDS education at levels below senior high school. School superintendents also note that many school districts give incomplete instruction or avoid it entirely (Ficklen, 1988), the latter also consistent with our findings. At the same time, it is encouraging that half of the states in the nation have mandated AIDS education and are involved in developing standards and curriculum materials for AIDS education. It is also heartening to note that various agencies and organizations have developed resource guides for teachers (e.g., United States Department of Education, 1988; Keough, 1988). Our data show that in numerous cases medical professionals collaborate with local school districts in developing such curriculum materials. Also encouraging is our finding that parents uniformly support the schools that offer education about AIDS. Concerted and coordinated efforts in curriculum development, in-service training, and community agencies and organizations are probably most successful in bringing about effective AIDS education for our children.

References

American Academy of Pediatrics Committee on School Health (1988). "Acquired Immunodeficiency Syndrome Education in Schools." *Pediatrics,* 82:278–280.

American School Health Association et al. (1988). "National Adolescent Student Health Survey." *Health Education,* 19:4–8.

Centers for Disease Control (1989). "HIV Epidemics and AIDS: Trends in Knowledge—United States, 1987 and 1988." *Morbidity and Mortality Weekly Report,* 38: 353–363.

Citizens Commission on AIDS for New York City and Northern New Jersey (1989). *AIDS Prevention and Education: Reframing the Message.* (121 Sixth Ave., New York, NY 10003).

Coalition of National Health Education Organizations (1988). "Instruction About AIDS Within the School Curriculum." *Journal of School Health,* 58:323.

Ficklen, E. (1988). "Report: Instruction on AIDS Is Spreading." *American School Board Journal,* 175:34.

Forrest, D. J., and Silverman, J. (1989). "What Public School Teachers Teach About Preventing Pregnancy, AIDS, and Sexually Transmitted Diseases." *Family Planning Perspectives,* 21:65–72.

Fraser, K., and Mitchell, P. (1988). *Effective AIDS Education: A Policymakers Guide.* Alexandria, VA: National Association of State Boards of Education.

Gallup, G. H. (1981, September). "The 13th Annual Gallup Poll of the Public's Attitudes Toward the Public Schools. *Phi Delta Kappan,* 63:33–47.

Kenney, A. M.; Guardado, S.; & Brown, L. (1989). "Sex Education and AIDS Education in the Schools: What States and Large School Districts Are Doing." *Family Planning Perspectives,* 21:56–64.

Keough, K. (1988). *Dealing with AIDS: Breaking the Chain of Infection: A Guide for Developing an AIDS Education Program.* Arlington, VA: American Association of School Administrators.

Kerr, D. L.; Allensworth, D. D.; Gayle, J. A.; and Dalis, G. T. (1989). "The ASHA AIDS Education Needs Assessment: Association for the Advancement of Health Education Results." *Health Education,* 19:16–20.

Kirby, D. (1980). "The Effects of School Sex Education: A Review of the Literature." *Journal of School Health,* 50:559–563.

____; Alter, J.; and Seales, P. (1979). *An Analysis of U.S. Sex Education Programs and Evaluation Methods.* Atlanta, GA: Centers for Disease Control.

Koop, C. E. (1986). *Surgeon General's Report on Acquired Immune Deficiency Syndrome.* Washington, DC: U.S. Department of Health and Human Services.

____ (1989). Address Presented to the Joint Session on AIDS of the California Legislature, Sacramento, CA: March 6, 1987. In I. B. Corless & M. Pittman-Lindeman, eds., *AIDS Principle, Practices and Politics. Reference edition* (pp. 197–203). Washington, DC: Hemisphere.

Lansford, L. (1988). "'Best' AIDS Education Program Goes Nationwide." *The Center,* Gainesville, FL: University of Florida Health Science Center, 3.

Louis Harris & Associates (1988). *Public Attitudes Toward Teenage Pregnancy Sex Education and Birth Control.* Poll conducted for the Planned Parenthood Federation of America (810 Seventh Ave., New York, NY 10019).

Presidential Commission on the Human Immunodeficiency Virus Epidemic (1988).

Report of the Presidential Commission on the Human Immunodeficiency Virus Epidemic. Washington, DC: U.S. Government Printing Office, 88–91, 125–126.

U.S. Department of Education (1988). "AIDS and the Education of Our Children: A Guide for Parents and Teachers." Washington, DC: Consumer Information Center.

U.S. Department of Health and Human Services, Public Health Service, & Centers for Disease Control (1988). *Understanding AIDS.* HHS Publication No. (CDC) HHS-88-8404.

____, ____, ____ and Center for Health Promotion and Education (1988). "Guidelines for Effective School Health Education to Prevent the Spread of AIDS." *Health Education,* 19:6–12.

Yarber, W. L. (1979). "Instructional Emphasis in Family Life and Sex Education: Viewpoints of Students, Parents, Teachers, and Principals at Four Grade Levels." *Journal of School Health,* 49:263–265.

Chapter Three

Confusion Regarding HIV/ AIDS and Sexual Orientation: Its Impact on the Public School System

Beth M. Rienzi
Daryl L. Hitchcock
A. Odasuo Alali

Acquired Immune Deficiency Syndrome (AIDS) has been a major health threat in the United States for at least ten years, yet it continues to be misunderstood by the general public. This medical issue has been misconstrued as a social issue because of a general fear of this disease. Needed resources have been inappropriately diverted while the public reaction has gone from denial of the problem to blaming of the victims. Effective intervention with this epidemic will require a greater understanding of the social fear of AIDS.

Fear of AIDS and Homophobia

The human immunodeficiency virus (HIV) found to be the cause of AIDS is present in all populations regardless of sexual orientation, but its being labeled as a gay problem adds to the negative sentiment already directed at gay individuals (Haaga, 1991). Fear of AIDS and homophobia have been linked by previous research, with some inconsistent gender differences. Bouton, Gallaher, Garlinghouse, Leal, Rosenstein, and Young (1987) found men to be significantly more homophobic than females, but found no significant gender differences for fear of AIDS. McDevitt, Sheehan, Lennon, and Ambrosio (1990), using different measures, found that men scored significantly more homophobic, but were also significantly higher on their fear of AIDS.

Homosexuality has been intertwined with AIDS, and gay individuals are often blamed for the epidemic (Poirier, 1988). The mass media have focused considerable attention and blame on the stereotypical promiscuous gay male. The result has been confusion and fear about the causes and transmission of AIDS.

Fear of AIDS as a Media Construct

It is common knowledge that the mass media, particularly television, provide a majority of Americans the symbolic environment that determines their world views. The media perform this role through news reportage, paid advertising, shows, and public service announcements. As key gatekeepers, the media help people to construct and interpret reality about health issues.

Dissemination of AIDS information in the media often revolves around four social dimensions (Alali, 1992): sensationalism, deviance, stigmatization, and innocence. The sensational angle is usually defined by the celebrity status or the personality involved in the AIDS story. Clearly, the plight of basketball star Earvin "Magic" Johnson and the AIDS-related deaths of actor Rock Hudson, tennis star Arthur Ashe, entertainer Liberace, and high-profile lawyer Roy Cohn are a few of the most sensational AIDS stories in mainstream media. To some extent, media coverage of Ryan White and other school-age children took a sensational angle.

While most media operatives would have us believe that the more widely the disease is acknowledged in the media, the more easily it can be accepted (Alter and McKillop, 1986), the truth of the matter is that most AIDS stories do not enlighten or educate people. Rather, they are media scoops that scare people. Media scoops and education do not mix.

Media association of AIDS with lifestyles that are labeled "deviant" helps to construct "reality" about the disease. This media approach is reflected in a column by conservative analyst George F. Will, in which the liberal press is blamed for not telling the whole story about AIDS for fear of being accused of discrimination. In his column, Will (1987, p. 11) says that the liberal press has "refused to clarify that the primary reason for the AIDS epidemic is that the rectum, with its delicate and absorptive lining, is not suited to homosexual uses." Undoubtedly, this perspective serves no useful purpose but to further stigmatize those who live alternative sexual lifestyles. This assumption is widely held by most conservatives and the religious right, as is discussed in the next two sections.

The stigmatized status of those at risk for AIDS—intravenous drug users (IVDU) and, especially, gay men—is reflected not only in hard news reportage, but also in obituaries. Peter Nardi (1990) found that

> Obituaries provide an excellent source for illustrating the thesis of the social construction of reality.... In the context of a stigmatized disease disproportionately affecting stigmatized groups, the language used to explain early deaths among young men reconstructs the causes in an attempt to distance the deceased person from the disease and the risk group, thereby perpetrating those very stigmas [p. 161].

More often, when the cause of death is AIDS, obituaries identify the deceased as having died of pneumonia, lymphoma, leukemia, meningitis, etc. (Alali, 1994). Nardi (1990) posits that these terms actually clue the reader about the cause of death, and perpetuate stigmas about AIDS and persons with AIDS (PWA): "As more and more people learn to decode the language, the obituaries ironically have the opposite effect of actually signalling AIDS as the real cause."

The fourth social dimension in media reportage is innocence. The stigma about AIDS and homosexuals is rarely applied to heterosexuals who are infected with the virus. In most news reportage and dramatic television shows, heterosexuals who contract the AIDS virus are portrayed as "innocent" victims.

Clearly, media coverage of AIDS reaffirms the stigmatized status of homosexuals, thereby creating confusion and fear within the general population. Albert (1986a) sums it best: "The media portrayals of AIDS reflect the confusion and ambiguity experienced by the society at large." Bates (1990) suggests that "It is easy to see why, even in 1989, more than half the Americans polled believed that AIDS is transmitted during anal intercourse even if neither partner has AIDS." These social dimensions in the media have created a second disease, "AFRAIDS."

When unprotected anal intercourse was identified as the highest risk behavior to pass along HIV, politically conservative and religious fundamentalist groups wanted to brand gay men and ship them off to concentration camps (Poirier, 1988). Gay men were seen as the primary participants in this behavior. Self-identified heterosexual men that engage in this practice have been ignored. Blame is primarily directed at those individuals who engage in sexual contact not consistent with the mandatory heterosexual model.

Political Conservatives, Homophobia, and AIDS

Homophobia has dominated the entire epidemic period and robbed the public of effective leadership. Conservative political leaders, who have dominated political decisions and resources, help perpetuate the problem. Bouton et al. (1989) analyzed demographic variables in relation to homophobia and fear of AIDS, and found that conservative people are more homophobic and fearful of AIDS than are liberal people.

Conservative Senator Jesse Helms authored a bill, not a law, that prevents the "CDC from using federal funds for anti–AIDS campaign that 'promote or encourage, directly or indirectly, homosexual activities.'" When New York Mayor Ed Koch accused him of callousness toward AIDS victims, Helms wrote a letter to the editor of the *New York Times* (November 12, 1987) saying that "Americans who do not want to risk being killed by AIDS have a clear choice and a safe bet available: Reject sodomy and practice morality. If they are unwilling to do that, they should understand the consequences."

In a column that appeared in the *New York Post,* conservative Patrick Buchanan argued that AIDS is nature's way of striking back at homosexuals. While Buchanan is far from being the patriarch of the conservative movement, his views that "homosexuals were a major public health threat" strike at the core of prevailing conservative political thought. The conservative Bush administration paid as little attention to the disease as possible, as did predecessor Ronald Reagan, who "did not publicly utter the word 'AIDS' until the Rock Hudson story broke" (Apuzzo et al., 1986). Media collaboration, Apuzzo et al. (1986, p. 126) argue, permitted Reagan "to go through an entire first term and a bitter election campaign without ever once being questioned about his administration's handling of the most serious health crisis within recent memory."

Religion, Homophobia, and AIDS

It is impossible to separate organized religion from the homophobic complex that permeates other areas of society. In short, there is no separation of church, homophobia, and AIDS. The Protestant religious affiliation is more homophobic and fearful of AIDS than any other religious affiliation. Those who attend church more frequently are more homophobic and fearful of AIDS (Bouton et al., 1989).

Baldwin (1988) identifies four major church groups that illuminate the relationship between religion, homophobia, and AIDS: the far right church groups, the uncertain middle church groups, the active middle church groups, and the far left church groups. Of these four, the far right church groups are the most vocal because they view AIDS as a "deserved punishment for violating divine laws." This is also echoed in a *New York Times* survey in which 60 percent of those who identified themselves as "moralists" said that AIDS was "God's punishment for immoral sexual behavior" ("AIDS and the Real Electorate," 1988).

Other less influential groups often mimic these dominant and popular fears. Members of fraternities and sororities, for example, are more homophobic and fearful of AIDS than nonmembers. However, if a subject has had an acquaintance with a self-identified homosexual individual, that person is less homophobic and fearful of AIDS (Bouton et al., 1989), thus suggesting that direct exposure and knowledge of these avoided topics can decrease irrational reactions.

The general phobic reaction to sexual pleasure or erotophobia, which is a legacy of our Puritanical past, also complicates our society's response to this epidemic. Ficarrotto (1990) found that erotophobic attitudes were significant individual predictors of homophobia. Sodomy was outlawed in 24 states and the District of Columbia long before the AIDS epidemic. It was labeled an abomination against the laws of God and man (Poirier, 1988). The term sodomy is not legally well defined, but is often stretched for legal situations to include oral and anal sex, or "anything that involves the genitals which frustrates the impregnation of the ovum" (Poirier, 1988, p. 468). This reaction is further exaggerated by the taboo regarding activities associated with the anus. Thus those who engage in activities that are not sanctioned by God and become HIV-positive are believed to be righteously punished.

Homophobia can also be viewed as a prejudice, or "an injustified negative attitude toward a group and its individual members" (Meyers, 1990, p. 332). Racism and sexism, two other forms of prejudice, provide another link to homophobia. Ficarrotto (1990) found that by combining the prejudicial attitudes of racism and sexism, their effect on homophobia was equal to that of erotophobia. Since both phobic and prejudicial attitudes can equally influence homophobic reactions, prejudicial behavior should be separated from phobic behavior when attempting to understand individual reaction.

Homophobia vs. Heterosexism

During the last five years, there has been a movement to drop the word homophobia entirely and replace it with a more clearly defined word such as heterosexism. Heterosexism, which combines prejudice and power, is a heterosexual bias placing a superior value on heterosexual acts over homosexual lifestyles (Greene & Herek, 1994; Neisen, 1990). The saturation of this basic assumption pervades almost every aspect of our culture to create an ingroup and an outgroup.

David Haaga (1991) examines how actions that are labeled homophobic are actually not a phobic reaction but rather prejudice based. Haaga breaks this down into five components: problematic emotion, judgment of emotion, problematic behavior, political agenda regarding target, locus of motivation for change (Haaga, 1991, p. 172). The primary distinction is between fear and anger. Phobic reactions are of fear and anxiety, whereas prejudice contains anger, aggressive acts, and justification of its discrimination. Haaga concludes that better terms to use are "anti-homosexual prejudice" (Haaga, 1991, p. 175) and heterosexism. These terms better describe the biases and behaviors listed above, instead of including them in a fear oriented classification.

A homophobic reaction is best described from a psychodynamic perspective as an unconscious conflict about one's own sexuality. This conflict is temporarily resolved by projecting unacceptable personal impulses onto others, such as gay men, lesbians, and bisexual individuals. This is different from prejudice in that it is internal fear or doubt, not external bias and behavior.

Physical Anxiety and the Fear of AIDS

The horror of this disease is well known, so a fear of physical illness and life-threatening disease may exaggerate fear of AIDS. Fear of AIDS can be divided into rational fear and irrational fear. Rational fear includes fears about getting the disease if proper personal responsibility is not taken. Irrational fear includes fear of talking to a healthy gay male or a person who is HIV-positive, for fear of contracting the virus. Good and Parker (1977) developed a questionnaire to measure worries about physical problems which should be related to fear of AIDS if the basis of social fear of AIDS is in fact the result of the more rational response of physical anxiety. This question has not previously been investigated.

The present study (Rienzi & Hitchcock, 1992) examines homophobia, fear of AIDS, and physical anxiety of the subjects. We expected to find a connection between fear of AIDS and homophobia, with men being more homophobic and fearful of AIDS than women as suggested by previous research. Physical anxiety may also predict fear of AIDS if the worries are of physical disorders, not homophobic-linked irrational fears. Homophobia and physical anxiety should be unrelated if they are independent.

Method

Physical Anxiety Questionnaire (PAQ), Attitudes Towards Homosexual Scale (ATHS), and the Fear of AIDS Scale (FOAS) were administered to 88 introductory psychology students (65 of whom were women). Eleven of the subjects declined to participate. There were 10 African-Americans, 8 Asian-Americans, 18 Hispanics, 37 Whites, and 3 who marked "other," with one subject not responding. The subjects had a mean age of 21 years (SD=5.52) and ranged from 17 to 42, with one subject not responding. The PAQ is the exact scale from Good and Parker (1977), as was the FOAS from Bouton et al. (1987). The ATHS included the Homophobia Scale (Bouton et al., 1987) and the following additional questions for greater reliability:

I would feel comfortable if I learned that my best friend of my same sex was homosexual.
I would feel comfortable working closely with a male homosexual.
I would enjoy attending social functions at which homosexuals were present.
I would feel nervous being in a group of homosexuals.

I would be comfortable if I found myself attracted to a member of my sex.
If a member of my own sex made an advance toward me, I would feel flattered.
I would feel comfortable working closely with a female homosexual.
I would feel at ease talking with a homosexual person at a party.

The PAQ is a true/false questionnaire, while the ATHS and FOAS were scored on a 4 point Likert-type scale (completely agree, somewhat agree, somewhat disagree, completely disagree).

Results

The *t* tests comparing men to women on their homophobia and fear of AIDS scores found no significant difference. The homophobia scale correlated with the fear of AIDS ($r = .67$, $p < .001$). The scores on physical anxiety did not correlate significantly with either the fear of AIDS or homophobia.

Discussion

The results supported the hypothesis that fear of AIDS correlates with homophobia, and also supports work by Bouton et al. (1987 and 1989), and McDevitt et al. (1990). We did not find that men were more homophobic than women, as previous studies have reported (Bouton et al.; 1987 and 1989, & McDevitt et al.; 1990), nor did we find that men were more fearful of AIDS than women (McDevitt et al., 1990). The disproportionately large number of women tested in this study likely reduced the possibility of finding a significant difference between men's and women's scores.

The fact that no significant correlation was found between physical anxiety and fear of AIDS suggests that people do associate AIDS with homosexuality, and that the fear of AIDS is less likely to be related to fear of physical disorder. This is an important relationship to examine, since we have to educate society not only about AIDS, but about homosexuality as well. As long as our culture equates homosexuality with AIDS, several negative scenarios are likely. Many people will react to all gay men and lesbians as if they were infected with AIDS. Conversely, HIV-positive individuals are likely to receive the self-righteous judgmental reactions that conservative and religious groups reserve for gay men or lesbians. It is important to remember that many in these groups are willing to cast this same minority out of society for their abominable acts against nature based on their belief that God is using AIDS to punish gay individuals (Poirier, 1988).

Further study needs to discern the causes of homophobia, whether irrational fear or social prejudice. When discrimination against the gay community is held under the broader term of homophobia, it is seen as an individual's irrational fear of homosexual behavior, and not more appropriately as society's pressure to the heterosexual behavioral norm. Gay men, lesbians, and bisexual individuals form the largest group still excluded from their civil rights (Haaga, 1991). Their struggle against prejudicial and discriminatory behaviors is similar to that fought by African-Americans during the 1960s. Since heterosexism is no different from bigotry, perhaps society can begin the slow process of change through cultural education.

Fear of AIDS and the School System

Public reaction to AIDS and the virus that causes AIDS has often been less than rational. Individuals have a tendency to simplify issues using time-saving stereotypes even though these stereotypes may grossly distort reality. This study points out that much of the emotional reaction to AIDS and HIV is confused with ignorance, misinformation, and unrealistic fear not only about HIV and AIDS but also about sexual orientation in general. Future studies will need to investigate these connections further.

We recommend education to reduce unrealistic fears of HIV and AIDS, and suggest that this education must include a more realistic approach to the diversity of sexual orientation. Many of the college students who participated in this study will become elementary and high school teachers in the future. The prejudicial attitudes found in this study are likely to influence their future interactions with HIV-positive students. Children who test HIV-positive are likely to elicit subtle and direct negative reactions from teachers. This is a frightening concept given the rejection, discrimination, and violence that the gay community continues to suffer in this country. We suggest that a more appropriate reaction to HIV-positive children is impossible if homophobia and heterosexism are not directly and simultaneously confronted.

Efforts to reduce prejudice against HIV-positive students may be ineffectual without discussion of attitudes towards the gay and lesbian community. Fear of AIDS appears to be enmeshed with the phobic and prejudical reaction to the gay community, which has long been denied and ignored by the school system.

Traditionally, the schools have attempted to address mutually exclusive contradictory issues. The school system is caught in an attempt to balance conformity with diversity. The schools are given the task of teaching children conformity to the values and laws of the dominant culture while simultaneously addressing individual needs. Special programs have been developed to address the needs of many small identified populations. There are special programs for individuals that are retarded, gifted, hearing impaired, hyperactive or special. Some of these defined groups represent only 1 to 3 percent of the student body population. Considerable money, time, and training continues to be invested in these small populations, but the gay and lesbian youth in our school system are completely ignored.

This ignored population represents from 10 to 20 percent of the student body and no doubt 10 to 20 percent of the school staff as well (Francoeur, 1991). Conformity demands have not been realistic for these individuals. The past emphasis on an overly narrow, rigid, and idealized vision of all children and staff conforming to the mandatory heterosexual standard is clearly dysfunctional. Children have not been able to change their sexual orientation with any greater success than they can change their skin color. It is therefore ridiculous to burden them with pathogenic rejection, prejudice, and discrimination.

Gay students in the university setting find the colleges to be unsupportive of them (Reynolds, 1989). These colleges are likely to be more liberal than high schools, and the students would be expected to be more mature. This assumption would leave little hope of acceptance for the gay and lesbian teens still in lower grade levels. In fact, this may explain the high rate of suicide for gay youths. Lesbian and gay youths are approximately 2 to 3 times more likely to kill themselves than their more accepted heterosexual peers (Francoeur, 1991). As many as 30 percent of all teen suicides may have to do with sexual identity issues (Hersch, 1991).

Since homophobia is correlated with the fear of AIDS, students who are HIV-positive are bound to feel the overlap of these prejudicial attitudes. Gay-bashing is only one of the particularly frightening expressions of these prejudicial attitudes. In a recent survey of 500 gay and lesbian students, 20 percent reported they had suffered a violent assault because of their sexual orientation (Hersch, 1991). Not only must the HIV-positive teen deal with feeling like a pariah, but the added defensiveness necessary to combat the homophobia can increase the pressure dramatically.

One factor that may contribute to this neglect is the general denial of the existence of homosexuality by school staff and by parents. Schools in more conservative areas often prefer their gay and lesbian employees to remain "in the closet" and thus pass as being heterosexual. This not only robs students of potential healthy role models of gay and lesbian adults but perpetuates the denial of differences in sexual orientation. Since contact with self-identified gay and lesbian individuals reduces homophobia and fear of AIDS (Bouton et al., 1989), schools are ignoring an important source of understanding and an important opportunity for education if they practice these heterosexist policies.

This heterosexism of the educational system is also evident in the sexual orientation "gag rule." School teachers and counselors are often forbidden to discuss gay and lesbian sexual orientation. This situation may fit the needs of the dominant (and one might even say coercively domineering) heterosexual culture, but it has often not met the needs of the gay youth. This policy is likely to make life more difficult for the HIV-positive youth as well.

Problems That Need to Be Addressed Immediately

One problem noted in our school systems is the general invisibility of gay and lesbian individuals, the gay and lesbian lifestyle, and gay and lesbian issues. Gay and lesbian teachers and personnel in the school systems often fear economic and social reprisal. They often choose to hide their identity and publicly live a lie rather than risk their employment and income. This can be a problem for them as individuals, for their friends and family, and for the students who are then robbed of positive role models. This silence is also an issue for the HIV-positive youth.

In summary, the school system can create a more accepting environment for HIV-positive youth by making the classroom a more accepting place for gay and lesbian youth. This can be done inexpensively by encouraging the visibility of gay and lesbian teachers who are already hired in the school systems. The visibility of gay and lesbian lifestyle, history, and literature also needs to be increased in school curricula, textbooks, required reading lists, films, and lecture material. In many cases, the students are now studying famous gay or lesbian individuals, but the orientation and lifestyle of these individuals are avoided.

References

"AIDS and the Real Electorate" (1988, January 24). *The New York Times.*

Alali, A. O. (1992). *Fear of AIDS as a Media Construct.* Unpublished manuscript.

____ (1994). "The Disposition of AIDS *Imagery in New York Times'* Obituaries." *Omega: Journal of Death and Dying*, 29(4):273–289.

Albert, E. (1986a). "Illness and Deviance: The Response of the Press to AIDS," pp. 163–176. In D. A. Feldman and T. M. Johnson, eds., *The Social Dimensions of AIDS: Methods and Theory.* New York: Praeger.

____ (1986b). "Acquired Immune Deficiency Syndrome: The Victim and the Press," pp. 135–158. In T. McCormack, ed., *Studies in Communications,* Vol. 3, Greenwich, CT: JAI Press.

Alter, J., and McKillop, P. (1986, August 18). "AIDS and the Right to Know." *Newsweek,* p. 132.

Apuzzo, V.; Fain, N.; and Bazelli, R. (1986). "Education and Communication: Enhancing Public Understanding and Fostering Disease Prevention," pp. 105–128. In R. F. Hummell, W. F. Leavy, M. Rampolla, and S. Chorost, eds., *AIDS: Impact on Public Policy.* New York: Plenum Press.

Baldwin, D. C. (1988). "AIDS and Religion," pp. 51–52. In R. F. Schinazi and A. J. Nahamias, eds., *AIDS in Children, Adolescents & Heterosexual Adults.* New York: Elsevier Science Publishing Co.

Bouton, R. A.; Gallaher, P. E.; Garlinghouse, P. A.; Leal, T.; Rosenstein, L. D.; and Young, R. K. (1987). "Scales for Measuring Fear of AIDS and Homophobia." *Journal of Personality Assessment,* 51(4):606–614.

____; ____; ____; ____; ____ and ____ (1989). "Demographic Variables Associated with Fear of AIDS and Homophobia." *Journal of Applied Social Psychology,* 19: 885–910.

Ficarrotto, T. J. (1990). "Racism, Sexism, and Erotophobia: Attitudes Toward Homosexuals." *Journal of Homosexuality,* 9(1): pp. 111–116.

Francoeur, R. T. (1991). "Gender and Erotic Orientation." In R. T. Francoeur, *Becoming a Sexual Person* (pp. 431–462). Ontario: Macmillan.

Good, L. R., and Parker C. C. (1977). "Physical Anxiety Questionnaire." In R. S. Aero, and E. Weiner (1981). *The Mind Test* (pp. 49–50). New York: William Morrow.

Greene, B., and Herek, G. M. (eds.) (1994). *Lesbian and Gay Psychology: Theory, Research, and Clinical Applications.* Thousand Oaks, CA: Sage.

Haaga, D. A. F. (1991). "Homophobia" *Journal of Social Behavior and Personality,* 6(1):171–174.

McDevitt, T. M.; Sheehan, E. P.; Lennon, R.; and Ambrosio, A. L. (1990). "Correlates of Attitudes Toward AIDS." *The Journal of Social Psychology,* 130(5):669–701.

Myers, D. G. (1990). "Prejudice: Disliking Others." In D. G. Meyers, *Social Psychology* (3rd ed.; pp. 331–366). New York: McGraw-Hill.

Nardi, P. M. (1990). "AIDS and Obituaries: The Perpetuation of Stigma in the Press," pp. 159–163. In D. A. Feldman, ed., *Culture and AIDS.* New York: Praeger.

Neisen, J. H. (1990). "Heterosexism: Redefining Homophobia for the 1990s." *Journal of Gay and Lesbian Psychotherapy,* 1(3):21–35.

Poirier, R. (1988). "AIDS and Traditions of Homophobia." *Social Research,* 55(3): 461–475.

Reynolds, A. J. (1989). "Social Environmental Conceptions of Male Homosexual Behavior: A University Climate Analysis." *Journal College Student Development,* 30:62–69.

Rienzi, B. M., and Hitchcock, D. L. (1992, April). "Fear of AIDS: A Measure of Homophobia or Physical Anxiety?" Paper presented at the meeting of the Western Psychological Association, Portland, OR.

Will, G. (1987, June 9). "Concerns for Discrimination Blurring Truths About AIDS." *The (Madison, WI) Capital Times.*

Chapter Four

HIV/AIDS Education at a Typical Urban High School: A Teacher Survey

FIDELIS EJIANREH

A national survey of high school students in the United States indicates that half of them are sexually active, or have had sex before age 16 for girls and 15.5 for boys (Centers for Disease Control [CDC], 1989). That adolescents are having sexual intercourse at earlier ages and with increasing frequency is the reality.

Consequently, most of the large school districts in the United States now support education to help young people avoid becoming pregnant or contracting sexually transmitted diseases (STDs) like the human immunodeficiency virus (HIV) that causes acquired immune deficiency syndrome (AIDS). In their curricula, these districts emphasize that abstinence from sexual relations is the most effective strategy for achieving this aim (Kenney, Guardodo, & Brown, 1989). There are no indices, however, to measure the effectiveness of these programs. What exactly are high school students being taught? How is it being taught? What are the success or failure rates of these programs?

Forrest and Silverman (1989, p. 65) offer supportive arguments in their analysis of what public schools teach about preventing pregnancy, AIDS, and STDs:

> The emergence of AIDS and the recognition that it can be transmitted through heterosexual intercourse (Koop, 1986) have undoubtedly changed both the frequency with which students receive sex education and the content of that teaching. Although the policies and programs of states and school districts are important guides, they provide little precise information about what is taught in the classroom.

Additional evidence from a 1978 survey of high school teachers (Orr, 1982, p. 304) and a 1982 survey of superintendents of schools (Sonenstein & Pittman, 1984, p. 19) suggests that the contents of sexuality education curricula vary widely across the United States.

The prevailing public concern about AIDS and the sexual adventurism of teenagers prompted the present assessment of the attitudes of those who interact with these adolescents on a daily basis—teachers and counselors. Additional motivation for this research is attributable to the dearth of literature in this area. This chapter will focus on six main areas:

- Specific contents of AIDS curriculum
- Should teachers provide AIDS education? To students of what age?
- Teacher training in AIDS education
- Length of AIDS education teaching experience
- Methodology and materials used in AIDS education teaching
- Teachers' overall evaluation of their AIDS education program

Methodology

A survey instrument consisting of a six-category questionnaire was administered to teachers and counselors at a local high school in the Los Angeles Unified School District. Each survey category contained specific, detailed questions; some categories had more questions than others. There were a total of 42 questions, including one that was open-ended ("What specific problems, challenges, and concerns are you confronted with in teaching AIDS education and prevention?").

The survey instrument was placed in the mailboxes of 100 teachers and counselors at the school; 32 teachers responded on time, constituting a 32 percent response rate (the average response rate for most surveys is about 40 percent). The fact that the survey was conducted during final examinations week may partially explain the low response rate.

The survey methodology had some limitations; it was pseudoscientific at best. Chief among the limitations was the small size of the sample. No preliminary survey was conducted on focus or pilot groups and therefore ambiguity with some of the questions may have been inevitable. Nonetheless, the survey served its purpose of gathering general preliminary information in the six category areas identified.

Another strength of this survey pertains to the geographical location and the ethnic composition of the school from which the data were derived. The school surveyed is located in Hollywood, California, a very urban location. At the time of the survey, it had a student population of about 2,500, of which 55 percent are Hispanic, 35 percent are white (mostly Armenian immigrants), and

2 percent are African-American, with the remaining 8 percent about equally representative of literally all cultures and languages around the world. More than 40 languages are spoken among the student population; most students (65 percent) are designated English as a Secondary Language, a fact that may be pertinent to some of the responses.

The teacher demographic profile is similar to that of the student body. The average age (not a survey item) of the teachers was 42. The gender ratio of actual respondents could not be determined, because personal information items were not included in the survey instrument. No such information was volunteered; however, the entire teaching and counseling staff comprised 65 females and 51 males. Approximately two-thirds of the teachers were born outside of the United States (a fact which may also shape the responses). Responding teachers may also have included those who did not teach health or biology, because teachers in all subject areas were surveyed. The average duration of teaching experience was 14 years.

Results

For simplicity, all "strongly agree" (SA) and "agree" (A) responses and "strongly disagree" (SD) and "disagree" (D) responses were considered as agreeing or disagreeing, respectively, with the specific item; unless it becomes significant to differentiate between both. The percentages of responses were rounded off to the hundredths.

Specific Contents of AIDS Curriculum The majority of the teachers agreed with most of the survey's statements in this category (see Table 4.1). Nine percent of the respondents disagreed with including self-esteem education in AIDS education curriculum, whereas 3 percent expressed no opinion. Eighty-eight percent of the responding teachers felt self-esteem education was an important component of AIDS education curriculum. On whether values/morals education should be included in HIV/AIDS curriculum at this high school, 9 percent of the responding teachers said they disagreed; 83 percent agreed, and 6 percent had no opinion.

There was significantly more discord on whether parents should have input in developing an HIV/AIDS education curriculum; although 75 percent agreed, 15 percent disagreed, and significantly, 9 percent had no opinion. This was the most divergent item in this category, and understandably so. Having parents of diverse cultural and religious backgrounds providing input into a curriculum as sensitive as AIDS education can make for a confusing, if not disastrous, program.

Should Teachers Provide AIDS Education? To Students of What Age? As Table 4.2 indicates, the majority of teachers (81 percent) are of the opinion that states should not have to mandate AIDS education before teachers provide

Table 4.1: Specific Contents of AIDS Curriculum

Statement	*Total %*	*SA*	*A*	*D*	*SD*	*NO*
1. AIDS education should include sex education information.	100	72	28	-	-	-
2. AIDS education should include decision making.	97	72	21	-	-	-
3. AIDS education should include communication skills.	100	69	31	-	-	-
4. AIDS education should include self-esteem education.	100	75	13	9	-	3
5. AIDS education should include information about risk behaviors.	100	91	6	-	-	-
6. AIDS education should include information about risk groups for AIDS.	100	75	21	-	-	3
7. AIDS education should include safer sex behavior.	97	75	19	-	-	-
8. AIDS education should include misconceptions about AIDS.	100	91	9	-	-	-
9. AIDS education should include how AIDS is transmitted.	100	94	6	-	-	-
10. AIDS eduction should include counseling and referrals.	100	75	25	-	-	-
11. AIDS education should include values/morals education.	100	59	21	3	6	6
12. Parents should have input in AIDS curriculum.	100	34	41	3	12	9

SA=strongly agree; A=agree; D=disagree; SD=strongly disagree; NO=no opinion

it. Similarly, 69 percent of the responding teachers disagree that AIDS education should be explicitly permitted by schools before teachers can begin it. A significant 28 percent of the teachers, however, expressed the opinion that the school's permission is required to teach about AIDS. This may be attributable to three factors: the lack of state and school district AIDS education guidelines, the significant number of new teachers (i.e., those with less than 2 years experience) responding to the question, and the probability that a significant number of the responding teachers were not health, biology, or science teachers (making

Table 4.2: Should Teachers Teach AIDS Education and at What Age Should AIDS Education Begin?

Statement	*Total %*	*SA*	*A*	*D*	*SD*	*NO*
1. We should teach AIDS education and prevention only if it is mandated by State law.	100	3	6	19	62	6
2. We should teach AIDS education and prevention only if schools it.	100	3	25	28	41	3
3. We should teach AIDS education and prevention on a teacher's own initiative.	97	3	22	44	25	3
4. We should teach AIDS education and prevention because it is the right thing to do.	100	59	31	3	-	6
5. We should teach AIDS education and prevention only in response to student questions.	100	-	-	50	44	6
		Ages (in years)				
		0–6	*7–10*	*11–12*	*13–16*	*NO*
6. At what age should AIDS education start?	100	25	34	34	6	-

SA=strongly agree; A=agree; D=disagree; SD=strongly disagree; NO=no opinion

them more likely to be unsure of whether or not school permission is necessary). The lack of state and school district guidelines creates uncertainty in the minds of some teachers, especially new teachers who lack tenure and would rather "play safe" with such a potentially explosive subject as AIDS education.

Table 4.2 also shows that although a majority of the teachers (69 percent) disagreed that teachers should teach AIDS education only by a teacher's own initiative, 90 percent were of the opinion that teaching AIDS education is the right thing to do. Interestingly, although the majority of teachers reported that state, district, or school mandates should not be necessary in order for teachers to teach AIDS education, they also disagreed that it should be left solely to the discretion of the teacher. Education about AIDS was recommended because "it is the right thing to do," although it is unclear whether this was interpreted to mean the professionally ethical thing to do or the morally correct thing to do. These issues should be explored in follow-up studies.

Table 4.3: AIDS Education Training for Teachers

Statement	*Total %*	*SA*	*A*	*D*	*SD*	*NO*
1. Those who teach AIDS education and prevention should undergo basic public health education training.	100	44	41	16	-	-
2. Those who teach AIDS education and prevention should be credentialed.	100	22	31	31	18	16
3. I am trained to teach AIDS education and prevention.	100	-	34	53	-	9
4. All teachers should be required to teach AIDS education and prevention.	100	9	18	37	25	3
5. Only health teachers should be required to teach AIDS education and prevention.	98	9	15	50	15	9
				Years		
		1–2	*3–4*	*5–6*	*7+*	
6. How many years have you been teaching AIDS education and prevention?	52	22	6	12	3	9

SA=strongly agree; A=agree; D=disagree; SD=strongly disagree; NO=no opinion

There was a clear lack of consensus as to the age at which AIDS education should begin (see Table 4.2). Of the responding teachers, 34 percent said that AIDS education should start at the elementary school grades (ages 7–10), 34 percent preferred the junior grades (ages 11–12), and 25 percent opted for the kindergarten grades (0–6). One teacher suggested fetal communication.

AIDS Education Training for Teachers Table 4.3 indicates that the majority of teachers were of the opinion that special AIDS education training should be provided for teachers. They were equally divided, however, on whether a credential should be required to teach AIDS education. Again, a possible reason for the large percentage of teachers who disagreed with this question could be the relatively large number of teachers outside the fields of biology and health responding to this item. Because these teachers would not normally teach AIDS education as part of their curriculum, they would therefore view the credential process as an unnecessary burden. Fifty-three percent

Table 4.4: Program and Material Selection

Statement	SA	A (Yes)	D (No)	SD	NO (NR)
1. My AIDS education and prevention lectures are augmented with guest speakers.	-	41	12	-	53
2. My AIDS education and prevention lectures are augmented with resources from community-based organizations.	-	37	9	-	56
3. My AIDS education and prevention lectures are augmented with workshops.	-	9	31	-	62
4. My AIDS education and prevention lectures are augmented with audiovisuals.	-	25	19	-	59
5. My AIDS education and prevention lectures are augmented with role playing and/or dramatization.	-	19	22	-	59
6. Uniform guidelines are needed to teach AIDS education and prevention.	25	66	6	-	6
7. AIDS education and prevention should be supplemented with peer education and/or counseling.	40	56	3	-	3
8. AIDS education and prevention should be supplemented with special events (AIDS awareness week, etc.).	47	50	-	-	6
9. AIDS education and prevention should be supplemented with a condom campaign.	37	40	9	-	15
10. AIDS education and prevention should be supplemented with brochures and handouts.	56	50	-	-	-
11. AIDS education and prevention should be supplemented with community-based interventions (speakers' bureau, guest lectures, etc.).	53	50	-	-	3
12. AIDS education and prevention should be supplemented with outreach activities.	44	50	-	-	9
13. At my school, AIDS education resources are available to students on demand.	25	53	3	-	25
14. At my school, parents play a role in what I/we teach students about AIDS education.	3	16	34	12	37

Statement	*SA*	*A (Yes)*	*D (No)*	*SD*	*NO (NR)*
15. At my school, there are appropriate teaching materials for AIDS education.	15	25	19	12	28
16. The present AIDS education at my school needs improvement.	19	44	9	3	25

of the responding teachers had not received any formal training in AIDS education or did not feel adequately prepared to teach about AIDS.

Although most teachers (62 percent) feel that not all teachers should be required to provide AIDS education, a similar proportion (65 percent) disagreed that *only* health teachers should do so. Interestingly, only 3 percent of the responding teachers had taught about AIDS in their classes for more than seven years.

Program and Material Selection Overall, Table 4.4 shows that most teachers augment their HIV/AIDS education and prevention lectures with guest speakers, community-based resources, audiovisuals, and so forth. Many teachers, however (31 percent compared to 9 percent who do), report not using workshops in their AIDS education program. Workshops simply are not commonly utilized as a classroom technique in high schools. Furthermore, a disturbingly high 22 percent of responding teachers did not use role playing as a teaching technique; only 19 percent reporting doing so. Role playing is a proven technique in pedagogy, and it is especially effective with students who have limited English-language proficiency.

The majority of teachers expressed a need for uniform guidelines for AIDS education and prevention, suggesting that no such guidelines presently exist. As shown in Table 4.4, most teachers believe that AIDS education and prevention programs should be supplemented with peer education and or counseling, special events (e.g., an AIDS awareness week), condom campaigns, literature, outreach activities, community-based intervention, and the like. A notable 9 percent and 15 percent of the teachers, however, disagreed or expressed no opinion regarding condom campaigns. The school where this survey was administered-participates in a district-approved condom program in which students can obtain condoms (plus abstinence and "safer sex" literature), no questions asked, from the school clinic and from designated teachers.

The survey indicated that 78 percent of the teachers have AIDS education resources available to students on demand. The specific nature of the resources was not included in their responses; the assumption is that these resources include audiovisual materials and the other survey items listed in Table 4.4. When asked if appropriate AIDS education teaching materials were available at their school, however, the teachers were about evenly split in their resources: 40 percent agreed, 31 percent disagreed, and 28 percent expressed no opinion. Even more confusingly, the majority of the teachers (63 percent) said the present AIDS education at their school needed improvement. This suggests that although the teachers are pleased with some aspects of the program, they also feel other areas need to be improved.

Asked if parents played a role in what teachers taught about AIDS, 19 percent agreed, 46 percent disagreed, and 37 percent had no opinion. (It is perhaps pertinent to mention that at the time of this writing, the Los Angeles Unified School District was embroiled in a controversy resulting from a recently board-approved Gay and Lesbian Pride Day observance. Many parents were infuriated and opposed any special recognition of gays and lesbians.) For the teachers who said parents played a role in their AIDS education program, it was unclear from the survey what the specific contributions of parents were. It could be surmised that parents played a passive role by being informed of what was being taught.

AIDS Education Program Evaluation Responses to the open-ended question, "What specific problems, challenges, and concerns are you confronted with in teaching AIDS education and prevention?" were scant but varied. With fewer than 45 percent of the teachers responding, issues of concern included apathy on the part of students, lack of parental consent to teach their children about AIDS and its prevention, lack of AIDS education information in languages other than English, and general misconceptions about transmission of the virus (HIV) that causes AIDS.

Teachers, often claiming that students felt infallible, expressed frustration about overall student apathy toward learning about AIDS. Typical comments included the following:

> Developmentally, they are not mature enough to recognize the consequences of their actions. "I'm not that kind of girl," "This is love, so it's okay" ... these are some of the resistant attitudes of AIDS education.

> Strongly held beliefs and misconceptions about who is at risk for AIDS. Teenagers' denial of the reality that they can get AIDS. Their overall reluctance to discuss their sexual behavior. Their reluctance to use condoms when having sex.

> Apathetic, inattentive students.

Some teachers complained about parental apathy and outright opposition to AIDS education. One typical statement was: "Some parents do not understand why their children should take AIDS education. Some students did not take AIDS education with me because their parents did not give them permission."

Others lamented a woeful lack of AIDS education and prevention material in Spanish, Armenian, and other languages to serve their large immigrant student populations. The following is representative of such comments:

> There needs to be more done bilingually—especially Spanish. There are too many Hispanic teen pregnancies. Something needs to be done to inform the latter community about AIDS in the heterosexual community....

Many teachers were concerned by student misconceptions about AIDS.

> I have found that some students believe they are not at risk or will be affected by AIDS. With this idea, they find materials [and] supplemental activities to be unimportant. Thus, it is very important to bring guest speakers ... who fall into the same group as these "interested" students.

A lack of AIDS education resources was also a recurring sentiment:

> Resources have become available. However, it would be *wonderful* for each school's health department to have a wide variety of materials available without having to worry about a search throughout the district for one important video!

Summary

This study shows that teachers want to teach HIV/AIDS education, and that most do. Many teachers are unsure of specific topics to be taught, however, or to what extent these topics should be covered. Teachers need clear, unambiguous state and or school district guidelines.

Tensions exist between some parents and teachers regarding the specific content of an AIDS education program. Some teachers (especially new teachers) either do not provide AIDS education or skirt around it for fear of antagonizing parents or school authorities. The majority of teachers believe parents should not participate in the development of the AIDS education and prevention curriculum. Even so, a partnership must exist between parents and teachers if the program is to be successful; teachers cannot effectively impart knowledge to students at the exclusion of parents. Parental reinforcement and encouragement of learned behaviors are necessary components of a successful program. Improved parent-teacher communication, organizing open houses or "back-to-school-nights," and providing general information about the school's HIV/AIDS education program may be helpful in reducing these tensions. Also, clear, supportive guidelines from states and school districts will be helpful.

Teachers do not agree as to the age at which HIV/AIDS education should begin. Some states, including California and Arizona, mandate HIV/AIDS education from kindergarten through twelfth grade (Durgin-Clinchard, 1991-1992, pp. 1–7). Certainly AIDS education ought to start before children become sexually active (e.g., about ages 7 to 9) in order to prepare them for what lies ahead. It is most important that children are taught early; the specific age at which such learning should commence is secondary.

Although teachers believe a special credential is not necessary to teach about HIV and AIDS, the majority say more training is needed. Education and AIDS awareness training could be provided in the form of workshops, guest speakers, college courses, and the like. School districts should provide time off, class coverage, and financial compensation if necessary for teachers attending workshops or engaged in awareness training.

This study suggests that there is a shortage of AIDS education materials, particularly in languages other than English. Commercial development of materials in Spanish, Armenian, and so forth would be valuable; making these materials available in the school library would also help. Identifying community-based sources of materials (county libraries, university libraries, foundations, etc.) is another possible key step.

The teachers in this survey are generally satisfied with their school's HIV/AIDS education program, but the study also shows that they feel the program still needs improvements. Teachers should individually and in groups, identify the specific areas for improvement and suggest methods for strengthening these areas.

In conclusion, the need to combat the spread of this dreadful disease requires educators, parents, and the community at large to coordinate their efforts in an effective manner to reach children early. Providing educators with interesting (*not* boring), accurate, informative (*not* propagandistic), and supportive (*not* threatening) HIV/AIDS education materials will be helpful in achieving this goal.

References

Centers for Disease Control (1989). *America Responds to AIDS: AIDS Prevention Guide.* Atlanta, GA: CDC.

Durgin-Clinchard, J. (1991-1992, December-January). "Silence Is the Voice of Complicity." *SIECUS Report,* 20(2):1–7.

Forrest, J. D., and Silverman, J. (1989, March-April). "What Public School Teachers Teach About Preventing Pregnancy, AIDS and Sexually Transmitted Diseases." *Family Planning Perspectives,* 21(2):65–72.

Kenney, A. M.; Guardado, S.; and Brown, L. (1989, March-April). "Sex Education and AIDS Education in the Schools: What States and Large School Districts Are Doing." *Family Planning Perspectives,* 21(2):56–64.

Koop, C. E. (1986). *Surgeon General's Report on Acquired Immune Deficiency Syndrome.* Washington, DC: U.S. Department of Health and Human Services.

Orr, M. T. (1982, November-December). "Sex Education and Contraceptive Education in U.S. Public High Schools." *Family Planning Perspectives,* 14(6):304–307; 309–313.

Sonenstein, F. L., and Pittman, K. J. (1984, January-February). "The availability of Sex Education in Large City School Districts." *Family Planning Perspectives,* 16(1): 19–23, 25.

Chapter Five

HIV/AIDS Education in Rural Schools

DORIS HELGE

The AIDS epidemic was first assessed in the early 1980s as an urban, gay men's health crisis. As time passed, urban intravenous drug users and hemophiliacs were found to have high and increasing prevalence of the disease. It is not difficult to understand how AIDS was viewed as a primarily urban phenomenon; the great majority of AIDS cases are indeed diagnosed in urban centers (MacDonald, 1989). Unfortunately, however, the perception that rural populations are somehow secure from the encroachment of the human immunodeficiency virus (HIV) is both erroneous and perilous. It is erroneous because AIDS has spread across the face of the nation. It is perilous because there seems to be a false security among rural populations, a belief of many rural citizens that "it can't happen here" (Castenada, 1992). It can and does occur across rural America.

In fact, recent studies have indicated a surge in AIDS across rural America (Painter, 1992). The National Commission on HIV/AIDS found a 37 percent rise in AIDS in rural areas, as compared to only a 5 percent increase in cities over 500,000 in population (*The Signal,* 1991; Loughlin, 1990). Rural America is ill prepared for the AIDS epidemic, both culturally and in terms of resources available.

Attitudes of denial are prevalent (Castenada, 1992; Painter, 1992; Helge & Paulk, 1989; Helge, 1991b). In many rural areas, "an epidemic of fear and bigotry is compounded by a shocking lack of health care access for AIDS patients" (Loughlin, 1990). In any event, AIDS is testing a rural health care system that is already struggling to survive. Stereotypical belief systems, inadequate HIV education, efficient communication grapevines in areas that lack confidentiality and anonymity, the threat of social stigma, and homophobia discourage high-risk individuals in many rural areas from being tested for AIDS and inhibit the treatment of HIV-positive individuals (Loughlin, 1990; Castenada, 1992; Helge & Paulk, 1989). Treatment is also inhibited by higher rates of poverty, inadequate health care systems, lack of government aid, and lower health care access, in general, among rural citizens. Some experts are now stating that rural teenagers in some geographic areas have higher rates of infection than teenagers in nonrural areas (Painter, 1992).

This does not mean that all rural, mainstream adolescents are necessarily at high risk for contracting HIV. The intent is rather to indicate that these young people do face a risk. Thus, rural schools bear a responsibility to take all appropriate measures to protect their youth from infection by this deadly virus. This means youth must be provided with medically accurate information concerning routes of transmission of HIV, and with the knowledge and skills necessary to prevent infection.

Availability of HIV/AIDS Education in Rural Schools

A 1988 study of 100 randomly selected rural school districts, funded by the Centers for Disease Control, was conducted by the National Rural and Small Schools Consortium (Helge & Paulk, 1989). The purpose of the survey was to gather baseline data on the number of rural schools providing HIV/AIDS education to their students; age and grade levels to which this education was presented; proportion of programs which were mandated by legislative action; goals of existing curricula and programs; and procedures used in evaluating outcomes of these programs.

A "rural" school district was defined as a school district located in a community with fewer than 150 inhabitants per square mile, or in a county in which at least 60 percent of the population resides in a community with no more than 5,000 inhabitants (Helge, 1981).

Survey questionnaires concerning the response of rural schools to the HIV/AIDS epidemic were sent to randomly selected rural schools in the United States. Fully 80 percent of the schools returning the surveys provided some form of HIV/AIDS education program. These programs varied greatly in goals, placement, length, and curricular content. A majority (56 percent) of schools with programs involved their communities in the development of these programs, and 90 percent permitted parents to excuse their children from HIV/AIDS education.

The most frequently named goals of these programs involved transmission of accurate HIV/AIDS information to students. A serious concern was the relative brevity of programs. Most programs were relatively short, with 59 percent lasting one day or less. Almost half (40 percent) were only 1–2 hours in duration, and only one-fifth lasted between half a day and a full day.

Schools were asked to report whether they included abstinence, condoms, safer sex, STDs, and homosexuality in their HIV/AIDS program, and to list any other topics they included in their program. The majority (72 percent) of all schools included abstinence, 55 percent included condoms, 54 percent included safer sex, 53 percent included homosexuality, and 74 percent included STDs in their program. Almost half of all schools, or 60 percent of schools with programs, included all five topics.

Fully 67 percent of schools reported that their HIV/AIDS education programs described specific behaviors that increased the risk of HIV infection. Almost two-thirds reported that their programs described abstinence from sexual activity and intravenous drug use as the only sure ways to avoid HIV infection. A lower, but still sizable, 42 percent reported that their programs described the effectiveness of condom use in decreasing HIV risk.

Schools were asked to give information regarding the placement and availability of HIV/AIDS education within their overall curriculum. Most frequently HIV/AIDS education programs were presented in the seventh and eighth grades (59 percent and 60 percent respectively), although many schools offered programs in several grades.

Almost half (45 percent) of the schools reported that HIV/AIDS education had been implemented as part of a more comprehensive school health education program. A total of 46 percent presented their program as part of a unit on sexually transmitted diseases. Over two-thirds of the schools reported that they provided at least some of their instruction within regular health classes. Over one-fifth reported providing instruction in their biology or science classes, and 14 percent provided instruction within their human sexuality classes. One-third of the schools held special assemblies or other programs for the presentation of HIV/AIDS education programs.

Most schools (72 percent) reported that their program was being taught by health education teachers. In addition, 59 percent of schools provided HIV/AIDS education to their special education students. Only 10 percent provided instruction in languages other than English, where appropriate.

A majority (60 percent) of schools included discussion of abstinence, condom use, safer sex, homosexuality and sexually transmissible diseases in their curricula. More HIV/AIDS education programs were provided in upper than lower grades, and the majority of schools with programs included these within their health classes.

Another serious concern was that of the responding districts that had HIV/AIDS education programs, only 34 percent had tools for evaluating them.

Schools were also requested to provide information on any non–HIV related risk reduction programs they offered. Almost all (89 percent) schools presented substance abuse prevention programs. Over half (54 percent) offered programs intended to reduce the risk of teen pregnancy.

Fewer than half (44 percent) of schools offered suicide prevention programs, and only 30 percent had dropout prevention programs. Only 28 percent had other risk prevention programs in place, including health education (9 percent listed) and counseling programs (4 percent listed).

Respondents who did not have alcohol/substance abuse programs and prevention programs related to suicide and dropouts noted desires to have such programs. Many participants also noted that they would like to offer other risk reduction programs, including self-esteem, decision making, goal setting, and improving family relationships, but lacked appropriate resources.

Asked which programs they would like assistance with, participants listed teen pregnancy, alcohol/substance abuse, suicide, and dropout prevention. A total of 17 percent listed other risk related topics, including other aspects of HIV/AIDS (2 percent), peer counseling, and parenting programs (1 percent each).

Many schools also provided related programs. For example, 89 percent had substance abuse programs, and 54 percent had pregnancy prevention programs. Most schools had policies relating to the attendance of HIV infected students, but most did not have policies relating to the attendance of infected employees. The majority (55 percent) of schools surveyed stated that they had a policy relating to attendance of employees diagnosed as having AIDS or being infected with HIV. However, 39 percent did not have such a policy, and 6 percent did not respond to this item on the questionnaire.

A majority of schools (52 percent) did not have a policy on attendance of employees diagnosed as having AIDS or being infected with HIV. Almost half (41 percent) of schools did have such a policy, and 7 percent did not answer this item. Over half (56 percent) of all schools surveyed reported that their administrators, counselors, and or nurses had received special training or attended workshops about HIV/AIDS.

The investigators concluded that the large majority of rural schools in the United States offered some form of HIV/AIDS education to their students. The goals, placement, length, and curricular content of these programs varied a great deal, yet there were several common themes. These themes included the provision of accurate information on HIV/AIDS, development of a realistic perspective toward the epidemic, and development of skills for prevention of HIV transmission to their students. A slight majority of schools with programs provided instruction on a comprehensive range of HIV-related issues, and a similar majority involved the larger community, in some way, in the process of planning their programs.

Problems included the relative brevity of most programs and a lack of instruments to evaluate program effectiveness in most schools. In addition, a significantly minority of schools in this sample either did not provide HIV/AIDS education at all, did not provide comprehensive educational programs, or did not involve the larger community, and parents in particular, in the planning of these programs.

Researchers were also concerned that districts that did not return the survey did not have HIV/AIDS programs and thus possibly had lower motivation to respond. Even of those returning the survey, a significant minority (20 percent) did not provide HIV/AIDS education at all. Program brevity and evaluative processes were serious concerns regarding those with programs. Many rural schools did not offer health education, and many only provided 1–2 hours per week of any type of health education.

Two-thirds of all U.S. schools are rural, and 75 percent are small. This is a sizable constituency located primarily in traditional, conservative communities that are not usually enthusiastic about sex education. National studies have consistently indicated that successful sex education must be long term, integrated into an ongoing curriculum, and holistic in nature (i.e., combined with self-esteem, decision making, assertiveness, and other training). In addition, for effective implementation, rural citizens, outreach agencies, social groups, and parents should be involved in program design and implementation. This survey identified an insufficient amount of involvement of the larger community, and especially parents, in planning programs.

National Recognition of Needs for Sex Education

The need for effective programs to delay sexual activity and to educate teens regarding the HIV virus has never been greater. More than half of America's high school students report having sexual intercourse by the end of the twelfth grade. According to Painter (1992), about 30 percent of all children have sex by age 15; about 70 percent by 18. Only one-third of sexually active boys always use condoms. Nearly two-thirds of sexually experienced girls have had at least two partners, and up to 5 percent of teens take intravenous drugs, making them more vulnerable to HIV (Painter, 1992).

In the United States teens under age 15 are 15 times more likely to give birth than their peers in any other western nation (Buie, 1987). Over 25 percent of female teenagers (over 1 million each year) have experienced pregnancy (Kenney, 1987). Rates of sexually transmitted diseases (STDs) are higher in adolescents than in any other age group. In 1988, Shalwitz reported that 2.5 million American teens, or 1 in 7, would be diagnosed with some type of STD (Shalwitz, 1988).

The role of child sexual abuse in HIV infection has only recently begun to be investigated. The rate of sexual abuse in America is growing rapidly, and some studies have found rural children at higher risk for abuse than nonrural children (Helge, 1991a, 1992; Sanchez, 1991). Child sexual abuse is directly related to teen pregnancy, the spread of the HIV virus, homosexuality, prostitution, drug and alcohol abuse, and other social factors related to AIDS. Increasing numbers of rural children are also running away from abuse and are becoming homeless. Homeless or abused children, particularly those engaging in "survival sex" to earn a living, are particularly vulnerable to sexual abuse and are particularly reticent to discuss their abuse (National Network of Runaway and Youth Services, 1991; Vanderbilt, 1992; Helge, 1992). Sexual abuse may also be the seminal event in the lives of HIV antibody positive adolescents and young adults. Thus, discovery of this underreported victimization can allow the process of intervention to begin (Dekker, 1990; Helge, 1992).

The problem is well recognized at all levels of the school system. For example, a survey by the Education Research Group reported that more than half of 716 administrators surveyed in a national study favored providing students with "birth control" as part of comprehensive school-based services. Yet 96 percent of U.S. school districts do not provide birth control, according to the survey. The vast majority of schools have not begun to develop comprehensive plans to deal with teen sexuality. School administrators simply have not wanted to broach a subject with such potential to inflame parents and communities.

In a recent national survey, school counselors stated that teen sexuality is part of the teenage lifestyle of risk-taking. Because sexual images and references are commonplace in today's society, educators view moral values as "crumbling" (Jolidon, 1989).

Parents also increasingly appreciate the need for schools to teach their children information concerning sexually transmitted diseases, including AIDS. In a recent Louis Harris poll (Harris, 1988), 89 percent of adults favored sex education in the schools. A full 73 percent supported making birth control information and contraceptives available in school clinics. (The percentage of adults who would support providing abstinence and birth control information is certain to be far higher.) Of course, these parents and many more also want their children to know that abstinence is the only completely safe form of AIDS prevention and to know what to do to avoid sex.

Students also recognize teen sexuality as a concern. Sexual issues were reported by 17 percent of junior high respondents in a national survey as their top concern, second only to drugs and alcohol (Sperling, 1989, p. 1-A).

The Relationship Between Teen Sexuality and Self-Esteem

The likelihood of a teenager becoming sexually active and engaging in high-risk sexual behavior has less to do with socioeconomic status than individual teens' values, goals, aspirations in life, and family environment. Teenagers (especially girls) who see a positive future for themselves are less likely to become sexually involved at an early age, and are more likely to use contraception effectively if they do have sex. In 1982, a Northeastern University study also identified a correlation between early parenthood and academic ability.

Older teenage females with poor basic skills were two and one-half times as likely to be mothers as those with average basic skills. Older teenage males with poor basic skills were three times as likely to be fathers. Among younger teens—those under 16—females with poor basic skills were five times as likely to become mothers as those with average skills (Kenney, 1987).

Teen sexuality is loaded with embarrassment, shame, fantasy, insecurity, urgency, external and often conflicting pressures, and other complicating factors. Thus, knowledge alone is generally not of much help in real life, spontaneous, emotionally laden situations. While only about 5 percent of teens are believed to use drugs intravenously (Painter, 1992), a majority do use alcohol or other chemicals which can impair judgment (Rotheram-Borus and Koopman, 1989). Keller et al. (1988) found that sexual activity and drug use were positively associated in a teen cohort, regardless of age. The recent increases in teenage drug and alcohol use in the U.S. indicate the potential societal effects of these statistics.

Many children who have been sexually abused engage in precocious sex or survival sex (prostitution). The characteristics of children who have been sexually abused range from model "people-pleasing" behavior to acting out sexually, suicide, violence, etc. Without intervention and treatment, there is a risk of low self-esteem and unsafe sexual practices.

All teens need real opportunities to grow into productive, self-sufficient adulthood. Only this will produce the motivation to delay sexual activity or to engage in only low-risk sexual behavior. Two of the most readily identified and important factors are education and employment opportunities. Although teen sexuality with high-risk behavior is a national problem affecting all races and all economic strata, data clearly indicate that low income and minority groups—which typically can offer their young people fewer opportunities—suffer the most severe impact (CDF Reports, 1986).

Problems with Existing Sex Education Programs

Jorgensen (1981) and Paulk (1989) cited a formidable array of barriers to the effectiveness of teen sex education. These include teens' own levels of cognitive development, traditional sex role perceptions, parental lack of involvement with educational efforts, and the negative effects of mass media on the sexual socialization of youth. In the face of these and other barriers, it is not surprising that most teen sex education programs have been shown to be, at best, minimally effective (Kirby, 1984; Zelnik and Kim, 1982; Paulk, 1989).

Few sex education resources address males, and none describe strategies for rural programs. When males are approached, it is usually from an intellectual point of view (e.g., information receiving) versus a behavioral or attitudinal point of view. According to the Men's Reproductive Center, the relatively few male-oriented projects across the United States usually have not lasted more than three years. Funding agencies typically either do not fund them or else prioritize care programs for pregnant teens and do not continue funding male-oriented programs.

Success Factors in Teen Sex Education Programs

Paulk (1985) found three factors which appear to facilitate the success of teen sexuality efforts. First, the program should be long enough to effect significant, lasting change. Second, the program should be comprehensive, dealing with as many as possible of the varied issues surrounding risk-taking. These issues include sexual and contraceptive knowledge, self-esteem, decision-making skills, and assertiveness skills. Finally, the program should involve students, intellectually and emotionally, in the learning process (Helge & Paulk, 1989).

Most teens wait one year after becoming sexually active before seeking medically supervised contraceptive care (Kenney, 1987). Shortening the delay between the first intercourse and use of effective contraception could significantly reduce the chances of teens contracting HIV.

Significantly impacting sexual risk-taking behavior is difficult, and designing and implementing effective programs requires commitment and creativity. Effective programs require prevention and care services involving every available and appropriate community agency. Male roles must be addressed in terms of sexual issues and contraception. Males and females must understand that to avoid contracting HIV, they must abstain from sex or use contraception consistently and effectively. Many youth will be most comfortable abstaining from sex. Others must learn the risks of sexual behavior, what to do to abstain or make sex safer, and how to manage social situations so that they can.

Studies have clearly indicated that youth who engage in open, frank communication with their parents (fewer than 15 percent of all adolescents) are more likely to succeed in delaying intercourse or having protected intercourse. The family life education these youngsters receive in schools, churches, youth groups, and medical facilities reinforce and enhance their knowledge of "safe" sexual practices. Youth service providers including doctors, nurses, therapists, probation officers, educators, coaches, and youth group leaders must continue to support and educate these young people while addressing the needs of the other 85 percent (Shalwitz, 1988).

Program planners must remember that the youth services providers are themselves heterogeneous. Some are comfortable discussing issues related to sexuality, sexually transmitted diseases and HIV infection, condom use, and drugs, and some find these topics unacceptable and disquieting. Therefore, each worker and agency must examine its scope and limitations in dealing with prevention. Workers must be continuously trained and supported.

The last decade's experience with sex education has glaringly revealed that didactic "one shot deals" are ineffective in changing behavior. Successful prevention strategies are most likely to succeed if the following components are included (Shalwitz, 1988).

- Information and messages communicated to youth must be accurate, brief, explicit, and direct as well as consistent and repetitive. Ambiguous and judgmental terminology such as "sexually active," "bodily fluids," and "promiscuous," should be avoided. Due to the serious nature of the material, humor and engaging presentations are often greatly appreciated. Messages may need to be articulated multiple times before being heard. Thus, service providers must be patient and tenacious.
- Youth will respond in a more positive and interested manner when they hear a message from a person they trust, whether it be a parent, friend, or counselor. Therefore, it is of utmost importance that service providers understand the social norms and values of the target population as well as their HIV-related risk factors. Activities and materials must be linguistically, culturally, educationally, and developmentally appropriate and sensitive. Audio-visual aids which represent the target population make the issues presented more believable and realistic.
- AIDS/HIV infection must be presented within the context of the broader societal/family life issues young people experience. Education must incorporate values clarification, self-empowerment, and skills development, particularly in the areas of communication, decision making, and assertiveness training. These features should be threaded through a comprehensive family life education scheme which should include but not be limited to the following: anatomy and physiology; sexual development; cultural values and norms; pregnancy, STDs, HIV infection, contraception; parenting; violence/abuse; substance abuse; racism and homophobia; and self-esteem. It is important to communicate the interrelationships of high-risk behavior and sexually transmitted conditions (pregnancy, sexually transmitted diseases, and HIV infection).
- Youth and parents should be incorporated into the design and implementation of activities and programs. Peer counselors, parent trainers, and indigenous outreach workers should be adequately trained and utilized wherever and whenever feasible, in schools and community-based sites. It is of utmost importance to capitalize on the positive power of peer pressure and support.
- All administrators and staff working with youth should be trained and educated at regular intervals regarding STDs/HIV infection, and other relevant issues. Staff should also be knowledgeable about the language and lifestyles of the youth with which they interact. Youth service pro-

viders should be given the opportunity to practice discussing these sensitive matters by role play and other methods.

- Educational and counseling activities must offer a flexible assortment of alternative methods, behaviors and options which achieve the primary goals of eliminating further spread of STDs/HIV infection. Activities will need to be modified according to the service site (e.g., schools, detention centers, 4-H clubs, grange clubs, extension agencies, etc.). There is not one standard "AIDS rap" that can serve as a model for information dissemination.
- Schools and or non–school-based prevention activities must be integrated into a comprehensive, coordinated service delivery system to youth. Appropriate and accessible medical, psychiatric, and support resources should be identified for the spectrum of youth who are low- to high-risk for HIV infection, uninfected, or diagnosed with AIDS. Ideally, these resources should have a primary interest in providing affordable, confidential, developmentally appropriate services to young people who are culture and language sensitive.
- Services sites or staff persons/clinicians who opt to disseminate condoms should never assume that a youngster knows how to correctly use them. Condom education, whether done individually or in groups, is more effective with a visual demonstration, using anatomically correct models rather than an oral presentation.
- Prevention and counseling programs should be evaluated for effectiveness and modified according to the latest information and the composition of the targeted population.

Why Teenage Sex Is Common

Studies have indicated that sex is not the main consideration in teenage dating. More important to boys is companionship and to girls is communication. Teens appear to have a difficult time separating sexual affection from other kinds of affection (*USA Today,* D-1, 1989a). It is essential that schools teach communication skills and the difference between intimacy and sex.

Clearly, the primary causes of teens' contracting the HIV virus include ignorance, poor sex education, poor school performance, depression, low self-esteem, being from an alcoholic or dysfunctional family or a broken home, lack of parental supervision, school adjustment problems (particularly early grade problems or transition problems from elementary to junior or senior high school), or being a school dropout (Samels, 1989). Child sexual abuse is also becoming recognized as a related factor (Vanderbilt, 1992; Zierler, et al., 1991; and Dekker, et al., 1990). Many of these factors are interrelated and some (such as poor self-esteem, living in a dysfunctional family, and poor academic performance) may be casual (Samels, 1989; Helge, 1988).

Sex Education, in Isolation, Is Not a Deterrent

The American culture is greatly influenced by the popular media—television, videos, movies, radio, and magazines. Most media vehicles promote sex as romantic and exciting but seldom address the responsibilities of sexual relationships, contraceptives, or the potential of contracting HIV. Many U.S. teenagers have been raised in single-parent households or in families in which both parents work. Many have been left to fend for themselves at an early age, and their role models are images they see on television and in videos. Many students are afraid their parents will think ill of them if they discover that they are using birth control. Thus, they continue to take unnecessary chances.

Researchers are also finally beginning to realize the particular difficulties faced by children who are being sexually abused at home. As this is experienced by one in three girls and one in four or five boys in America (Vanderbilt, 1992; Children's Safety Network, 1991; Winters, 1985; National Center on Child Abuse and Neglect, 1991), the implications are profound for the incidence of HIV. The fact that many schools are now initiating child sexual abuse prevention and treatment programs will have some effect, but many states have poor mandates regarding this, or none at all, and great damage has already occurred to children who have been abused (Helge, 1992).

Sex education is not a sure deterrent to teenage sex or teens contracting HIV. Research has repeatedly shown little correlation between participation in a unit on sex education and the level of teen sexual activity (Buie, 1987). Simply incorporating a unit on HIV education into other coursework may increase students' knowledge, but it rarely changes behavior (*USA Today,* D-1 & D-2, May 16, 1989). Rather than a one or two week session in high school, HIV education must be expanded to become, instead, part of a 12-year learning program with a broader agenda that includes encouraging young people to set long-term goals and to think beyond the present.

Research has clearly indicated that school sex education programs do not lead teens to delay sex, use birth control, or avoid pregnancy. Teens' sexual mores are molded instead by television, films, music, advertising, peers, and adult models (*USA Today,* D-1, April 1989). Schools typically offer, at most, a few weeks of scattered sex education lessons, and the majority of those teaching these lessons are not qualified personnel. Because sex is not an isolated behavior, effective sex education must be part of an overall health approach (Painter, 1989, p. D-1). Classroom programs must be supplemented by community-based efforts involving parents, churches, youth groups, and the media.

Early sex education programs and intervention can persuade sexually inexperienced students to postpone sexual activity. However, students who are already sexually active by the time they begin receiving sex education are unlikely to change their behavior or to use contraceptives more frequently as a result of the instruction (Geiger, 1992).

Unlike traditional sex education programs, one experimental curriculum called "Reducing the Risk" taught students how to resist peer pressure to have sex and encouraged them to visit stores and clinics to get information about birth control. According to the study, students in the experimental group consistently knew more about contraception 18 months after the program ended than did students in the control group. This knowledge, however, did not affect their behavior; sexually active students in both groups were about equally likely to engage in unprotected intercourse, the study found. However, at the 18 month mark, 24 percent fewer students in the experimental group than in the control group had begun sexual activity. Exposure to the curriculum also reduced by 40 percent unprotected intercourse among low-risk students and students who were sexually inexperienced when the program began. The researchers also noted that the program, which was considered controversial in some of the communities that included it, did not increase sexual activity among teenagers. "It may actually be easier to delay the onset of intercourse than to increase contraceptive practice" (Geiger, 1992).

Problems Specific to Rural Areas

Two-thirds (67 percent) of U.S. schools are rural. According to a number of surveys (*USA Today,* D-1, January 20, 1989; Jolidon, 1989), rural teens are as sexually active as their nonrural peers. Yet rural schools are the least likely to offer HIV education to their students. Frequently, rural communities with traditional value systems resist sex education. Schools which do provide it frequently lack appropriate curriculum or resources to secure instructional materials. Many rural school districts lack qualified health educators or other teachers who are comfortable with sex education and being known as the community "sex educator." Many rural schools do not offer health education, and those that do frequently limit it to 20–40 minutes per week. Because of this time limitation and community resistance to sex education, it is not usually integrated into health education as it typically is in nonrural schools.

Even with HIV education mandated by many states, rural sex education is typically minimal. For example, the national survey reported earlier in this chapter indicated that while a majority of respondents stated that their schools provided some form of mandated HIV education, 90 percent permitted parents to excuse their children from this education (Helge & Paulk, 1989). Most programs (59 percent) took place in one day or less, and most HIV education programs were provided in upper rather than lower grades. Thus, sex education was of an even shorter time span than in many nonrural areas although it was oriented specifically toward HIV education because of state mandates (Helge & Paulk, 1989). The survey indicated that most of the programs did not meet the criteria described earlier as essential for an effective sex education program.

The prevalence of at-risk students in rural areas of the United States is high (Helge, 1991a; Geiger, 1992; Sanchez, 1992). Rural areas typically have disproportionate percentages of students from poor families. Many rural communities are composed of Hispanic migrants and other non–English speaking populations or other minorities such as southern African-Americans and Native Americans. Many of the factors associated with teens' contracting HIV such as poverty, dysfunctional families, poor economy, isolation, alcoholism, lack of parental support, high dropout rate, low student and adult aspirations, low peer and parental expectations, child abuse, lack of economic opportunities, and limited available social activities, are more prevalent in rural areas (Helge, 1991b; 1988).

Child sexual abuse is frequently overlooked in communities in which confidentiality of reporting is virtually nonexistent. In such areas, a job may depend on not offending a child abuser and counseling services may be inadequate. The prevailing attitude may be "family business is family business," and there may be a lack of knowledge that reporting of abuse is a legal requirement.

Successful role models, particularly female, are frequently difficult to find. There is typically little or no qualified counseling concerning personal development issues or individual counseling concerning sexual issues. Health and mental health resources are frequently absent in rural areas, particularly those that are geographically remote or isolated. Community mental health resources are also inadequate, and the majority of rural schools do not employ school counselors, primarily for financial reasons. Psychologists and counselors, when available, frequently spend a majority of their time conducting standardized tests or designing class schedules, rather than counseling individual students or groups (Helge, 1988).

Sexual activity frequently begins in elementary school, especially in impoverished areas. Rural schools do not have the resources of urban and suburban high schools for school-based programs (e.g., family planning clinics). Traditional rural attitudes generally prohibit this. In fact, data collected from rural schools field-testing HIV education curriculum modules for the National Rural and Small Schools Consortium HIV education project indicated that they only selected curricula that were "appropriately traditional, conservative, and emphasized abstinence." Most rural districts were offering sex education only because of state HIV education mandates.

A majority of rural communities do not have planned parenthood and related agencies geographically accessible to them. Youth-serving agencies such as boys' clubs, YWCAs, and YMCAs are nonexistent in many rural communities. Established agencies such as cooperative extension (county agricultural agencies) or 4-H clubs are generally not tapped by schools as rural sex education resources. Male reproductive health resources are virtually unknown in rural America.

Most grants or other programs available to rural areas emphasize services to pregnant teens over sex education or AIDS prevention. Research regarding school-based clinics that provide birth control have revealed a decline in teenage pregnancy (Painter, 1989, p. D-1). Such clinics follow an urban model. There are simply not enough students in sparsely populated, isolated rural areas to merit such an approach. In fact, a comprehensive literature review revealed that most innovative pregnancy prevention projects are city-oriented and are not easily adaptable for sparsely populated rural areas. Examples of innovative programs include New York City and New Orleans' traveling theaters, and Oakland's programs of meeting boys at major sports events and taking them to planned parenthood clinics. While the National Urban League sponsors programs in more than 70 cities to prevent and deal with teen sexuality and over 100 schools across the United States have school-based clinics, rural areas lack such programs.

Rural HIV Education

Programs tailored for HIV education in rural areas are definitely needed. Strategies for creating any type of change in rural areas are best implemented by local personnel who feel that the change is at their initiation or that it at least addresses a perceived need of theirs. Significant change will most likely occur with approaches that are holistically and experientially based and that take the time to process information, as opposed to those that assume that cognitive "one shot" curriculum approach will produce results.

As reported by Lloyd Kolbe of the Centers for Disease Control (*USA Today,* D-2, May 16, 1989), even though national surveys have clearly indicated that teens know the basic facts about AIDS, they are not doing much to protect themselves. If it is to be effective, HIV education has to be more than information transmission. It must include decision making, communication skills, and self-esteem education. Students with high self-esteem will care enough about themselves and others to make decisions to improve their future rather than unnecessarily place themselves at risk.

It is clear that self-esteem education must be integrated with HIV education. This cannot occur within a few hours. This design is necessary so that students have both the strength and the knowledge to abstain from early sex or, at least, to practice safer sex. Accomplishing this in conservative, under-funded rural schools is an exciting challenge.

Approaches to HIV education that will be successful in rural areas will include curriculum palatable to local community values and mores, sex education support from local community organizations and parents, educational approaches consistent with community values, alternate social activities and reward systems for teens, qualified sex educators or other teachers who are comfortable with sex education and with being known in the community as a sex educator, and successful role models.

Successful program planning will account for the fact that rural communities are extremely heterogeneous depending on their economic base and social cultures. Approaches to be used must incorporate career counseling, vocational training, and involve churches, parents, youth groups, and the media. Rural communities do have a number of unusual resources that generally have not been effectively used. For example, since citizens in small, rural communities typically care about each other and neighbors help neighbors, extended families and existing outreach systems should be used. This would include the cooperative extension service (county agricultural agencies), 4-H club, public health educators, and outreach personnel such as bookmobile staff, mail carriers, and meter readers.

An illustration of the unique strategies required to implement HIV education in rural schools is the involvement of county extension personnel. They are "out and about" in the local community, know everyone, and are selected for their positions because they are respected citizens and thus listened to. Other examples of parties to be educated and involved for effective HIV education programs are extended families (more prevalent in rural areas), and other "natural outreach providers." These providers may include public health agency personnel, meter readers, mail carriers, bookmobile personnel, and others who are effective communicators with the population they serve. The local communication and power structures must be acknowledged and effectively used. For example, the one gas station attendant in a remote rural area talks to lots of folks each day and can change opinions. The clerk at the one grocery store in a rural area is another resource.

Most such individuals, according to National Rural and Small Schools Consortium and American Council on Rural Special Education on-site studies, are well respected in the local community and can make or break a project. It is also critical to involve local social organizations no matter how few and how small they may be. For example, the garden club could show a Red Cross HIV education film as a program. The 4-H club, a county extension meeting, the Grange organization, VFW, and local churches could do the same. Any social organization, informal or formal, can be a vehicle for implementing HIV education. If rural citizens perceive the project as relevant to the community and if they are involved in designing and implementing the project, it will be more likely to be implemented. Such groups are essential for school HIV education programs to be successful.

A Rural Model

Neither schools nor parents can solve the teen HIV/AIDS education problem alone. The first step will be the community's acknowledgment that HIV/AIDS is a community-wide problem requiring a community-based solution.

A key facilitator—a highly motivated individual or organization—must be identified and accepted by the community's critical communication and power sources and by school personnel. This person must receive any sex education training necessary for the individual to feel confident in the role and comfortable with discussing sexual issues and other topics related to HIV/AIDS education.

Information for the community's project development should be gathered, including the rates of HIV and AIDS, sexual abuse, school dropouts during a recent time period (e.g., ten years), drug and alcohol abuse, and the number of school dropouts that were teen parents. (The facilitator should keep in mind that nationally, 40 percent of all school dropouts are teen parents.) Key community groups should be informed of statistics such as the fact that for every teenager above age 15 giving birth, statistically there have been two pregnancies; for every teen below age 15 giving birth, there have been three pregnancies. Most teenage pregnancies are unreported (Adams, 1989).

Community resources for planning and implementation should be identified. A highly motivated planning group should be selected, and most of these members should be volunteers. This group should meet as frequently as necessary to identify its goals for the project and to emphasize that the project is a community-wide priority. Local news media and natural communication systems in the local rural areas should be used to publicize relevant activities of this group and its enthusiasm about the project. Meetings of the planning group should be open, and community members who are not officially part of the group should be invited to attend and give suggestions. Their input should be considered by the group in a format that will facilitate total community involvement or at least support for the project.

The community should compare its existing resources and services to "model" resources and services. This model will involve goal setting by the planning group. The goals or standards for performance of the program will be developed after reviewing such models. These activities will assist in pulling together community resources. Goals of the planning group should include designing a coordinated unified system that responds to a teenager's needs individually and confidentially.

The planning group should also design a process whereby students who are at a higher than average risk for drug and alcohol abuse or sexually transmitted diseases are identified at an early age (at least by junior high school). This should be done by a nonjudgmental process. All efforts should be made to protect the confidentiality of information about the teenagers involved and their families.

The committee's identification of students as highly "at-risk" should be objective. Students that should be considered include those who have involvement with crime, substance abuse, frequent depression, child abuse, poverty, dysfunctional or alcoholic families, and illiteracy. Students who are migrant workers, school dropouts, or who are both minority and poor should be considered. Discussions surrounding identification of such students should always be prefaced with the comment that across America, a vast majority of teenagers are sexually active and an average of one in four or five children is sexually abused. Additionally, high percentages of teens experiment with drugs and alcohol. Thus, all teenagers are statistically at risk for HIV and AIDS. Community resources should be assessed including counseling; education; health, planned parenthood, and related social services; volunteer group activities; career counseling; vocational training; sex education; and any school sex education programs.

Other community resources to be identified should include relevant local clubs or youth organizations, rural outreach agencies (e.g., county agricultural agencies, public health educators, 4-H club), interested nonjudgmental parents, and churches. Community planning should specifically detail approaches to be taken by the schools and all of the organizations identified. Curricular materials and other information and methodologies should be infused into ongoing educational, social, and spiritual development activities. Individuals and agency personnel who will be involved should be trained and should give and receive peer feedback regarding their abilities to be nonjudgmental and effective with teenagers. Individuals and agency personnel to be involved should be familiarized with all available community resources, model programs, curricular materials, and other information and methodologies.

As educators in rural settings have typically resisted sex education, this role should not be thrust upon them. It is perfectly acceptable for the local community planning group or its facilitator to tell educators that it is understood that their job descriptions do not typically include sex education and that they may not be comfortable with a sex education role. On the other hand, they need to understand that teenage sexual activity is affecting their ability to educate students and potentially endangering the community.

School personnel should be allowed to perform roles that are comfortable to them, and community resources should be recruited to assist with other HIV/AIDS prevention roles. For example, teachers can use their established relationships with students to welcome to the classroom visitors who will discuss topics with which the teacher is uncomfortable. These visitors might include teen parents, teen addicts who are in recovery, other parents, therapists, regional planned parenthood agency personnel, ministers, public health workers, doctors, and others.

Educators need to understand that they are not expected to be therapists and that it is understood that they have not been trained to conduct therapy. On the other hand, lists of competent mental health professionals should be made available so that they can lead individual or group discussions with students regarding the psychodynamics of adolescent choices. For example, it should be openly discussed with teenagers that sexuality is viewed by our society as a rite of passage into adulthood and that getting pregnant may be seen by the teenager as part of becoming an adult. Honest discussions also need to occur regarding sexually transmitted diseases and child sexual abuse. Dialogue should acknowledge the fact that some teenagers subconsciously try to become pregnant so that they are not faced with their uncomfortable fears about growing up and becoming responsible.

A critical point is that school personnel should be reinforced for what they do well and know that community resources are available to perform functions which they are not trained, comfortable, or motivated to accomplish.

Program implementation should be publicized in a positive way on an ongoing basis. Formative evaluations should be planned as all program activities are designed. Evaluation should be implemented so that the program can make necessary modifications on an ongoing basis. The total effort should be seen as an experience that is developmental, and evaluations should be viewed as essential to the program. The evaluation methodology should be consistent with the model resources and services discussed early in the planning of the program.

Conclusion

The virus that causes AIDS is spreading at an alarming rate across rural America, and rural schools and communities are not effectively dealing with the social and other effects of this problem. Community-based solutions that are comprehensive and holistic in nature will prevent many factors related to HIV and AIDS (e.g., sexual abuse, drug and alcohol abuse, and teen pregnancies). Rural communities must develop school-community partnerships to design community-specific responses consistent with local needs, values, and resources. The use of all informal and formal community resources unique to that particular rural community will strengthen community recognition of the problem and commitment to the solutions designed by local citizens and agencies. Comprehensive efforts designed to enhance student self-esteem and to provide sex education; career, health, academic and mental health counseling; HIV/AIDS education; alternate social activities, and facilitation of parent-child communication will assist in the prevention of AIDS. Efforts to stem child sexual abuse are also essential. These efforts will strengthen the physical, mental, and economic health of the rural community involved. The project planning and implementation process itself will strengthen the sense of community.

References

Adams, G.; Adams-Taylor, S.; and Pittman, K. (1989). "Adolescent Pregnancy and Parenthood: A Review of the Problem, Solutions, and Resources." *Family Relations,* 38:223–229.

"The Broader Challenge of Teen Pregnancy Prevention" (1986, September). *CDF Reports,* 8(5):1, 6, 8.

Buie, J. (1987). "Teen Pregnancy: It's Time for Schools to Tackle the Problem." *Phi Delta Kappan,* 68(10):737–739.

Castenada, C. (1992, February 17). "Students Stung by HIV Stigma." *USA Today,* A-3.

Children's Safety Network (1991). "A Data Book of Child and Adolescent Injury." In *Maternal and Child Health.* National Center for Education: Washington, D.C.

Dekker, A. H.; Earl, D.; McKeigue, J. T.; Aguila-Manalo, M.; Torres, H.; and Ahart, S. (1990). "The Incidence of Sexual Abuse in HIV Infected Adolescents and Young Adults." *Journal of Adolescent Health Care,* 11(3).

Geiger, K. (1992, January 15). "The Forgotten America. Schools and Development in Rural Areas." *Education Week,* XI(17):p. 4.

Helge, D. (1984). "The State of the Art of Rural Special Education." *Exceptional Children,* 50(4):294–305.

____ (1988). "Serving At-Risk Students in Rural America." *Teaching Exceptional Children,* 20(4):16–18.

____ (1991a). "At-Risk Students—A National View of Problems and Service Delivery Strategies." *Rural Special Education Quarterly,* 10(4):31–38.

____ (1991b). "Needs of Rural Schools Regarding HIV Education." *Human Services in the Rural Environment,* 14(3):25–30.

____ (1992). "Educating the Homeless in Rural and Small School District Settings." In J. Stronge, ed., *Educating America's Homeless Children and Youth: Policy and Practice.* Newbury Park, CA: Sage.

____ and Paulk, J. (1989, April). *HIV/AIDS Education in Rural Schools in the U.S.: Enough of the Right Stuff?* (Report of a study funded by the Centers for Disease Control), pp. 1–13.

Jolidon, L. (1989, June 9–11). "Not Easy at All." *USA Weekend,* pp. 6–7.

Jorgensen, S. (1981). "Sex Education and the Reduction of Adolescent Pregnancies: Prospects for the 1980s." *Journal of Early Adolescence,* 1(1):38–53.

Keller, S. E.; Schleifer, S. J.; Bartlett, J. A.; and Johnson, R. L. (1988, December 20/30). "The Sexual Behavior of Adolescents and Risk of AIDS." *JAMA,* 260(24):3586.

Kenney, A. M. (1987). "Teenage Pregnancy: An Issue for Schools." *Phi Delta Kappan,* 68(10):728–736.

Kirby, D. (1984). *An Evaluation of Programs and Their Effects: Executive Summary.* Santa Cruz, CA: Network Publications.

Loughlin, S. (1990, September 30). "AIDS Threat Becoming Real to Rural America." *Daily News* (Washington, DC).

MacDonald, Pen. (1989, May). "Where Are We Headed: Five Years from Now?" Presentation at Washington Superintendent of Public Schools Youth at Risk HIV/AIDS Workshop.

National Center on Child Abuse and Neglect (1991). *Child Abuse Digest.* Tampa, FL: Winters Communications, Inc.

National Network of Runaways and Youth Services (1991). *Runaway, Homeless and Other Youth in High-Risk Situations in the 1990s.* Washington, D.C.

Painter, Kim. "AIDS Grants Go to Private M.D.J." (1989, April). *USA Today,* p. D-1.

____. "Teaching Kids a Lesson About AIDS" (1989, May 16). *USA Today,* pp. D-1, D-2.

____. (1992, February 17). "AIDS Is Making Inroads Among Teens." *USA Today,* D-1.

Paulk, Jonathan (1985). *Comparison of the Effects of Confluent vs. Traditional Contra-*

ceptive Education on Young People's Knowledge, Attitudes, and Behaviors. Doctoral dissertation, University of California.

____ (1989, May). "Recommendations for High Risk Prevention Programming in Washington Region 3." Washington Region 3 HIV/AIDS Service Network Document.

Rotheram-Borus, M. J., and Koopman, C. (1991). "AIDS and Adolescents." In R. Lerner, A. C. Peterson and J. Brooks-Gunn, eds. *The Encyclopedia of Adolescence.* New York: Garland Press.

Samels, M. (1989). *Some Girls.* (Film No. VHS9062). Boston, MA: Fanline Productions.

Sanchez, S. (1991, December 18). "Double Dose of Bad News for Kids." *USA Today,* A-3.

Shalwitz, J. (1988). *AIDS/HIV Infection Prevention and Education.* Unpublished manuscript. San Francisco, CA: Dept. of Public Health.

The Signal (1991, January). Everett, Washington.

Sperling, Dan. "Sex Survey No Help in AIDS Fight" *USA Today,* p. A-1.

Vanderbilt, H. (1992, February). "Incest. A Chilling Report." *Lear's,* 4(12).

Winters, R. (1985). *Child's Abuse Digest.* Tampa, FL: Winters Communications.

Zelnik, Melvin, and Kim, Young (1982, May-June). "Sex Education and Its Association with Teenage Sexual Activity, Pregnancy, and Contraceptive Use." *Family Planning Perspectives,* 14(3):117–119, 123–126.

Zierler, S.; Feingold, L.; Laufer, D.; Velentgas, P.; Kantrowitz-Gordon, I.; and Mayer, K. (1991). "Adult Survivors of Childhood Sexual Abuse and Subsequent Risk of HIV Infection." *American Journal of Public Health,* 81(5):572–575.

Chapter Six

HIV/AIDS Curriculum Implementation in Rural Schools: Barriers and Successes

JAMES T. GIRVAN
LARRY D. FARRELL

The first cases of AIDS in the United States were reported in 1981 (Centers for Disease Control, 1981). By the end of 1991, a total of 206,392 cases of AIDS had been reported in the United States (Centers for Disease Control, 1992), and as early as 1987 many people considered AIDS to be the nation's most serious health threat (Stout, 1987).

Dr. Mervyn Silverman recently suggested that the United States is at a crossroads in the AIDS epidemic, stating that "The disease, those affected, their caregivers, the institutions—everything is changing" (Silverman, 1990). During the early days of the HIV/AIDS epidemic in the United States, most of the cases were reported in major urban areas. However, that pattern has changed significantly as the virus has continued to spread through the population. While the total number of AIDS cases reported in the United States between March 1989 and February 1990 increased 12 percent over the total reported during the same time period a year earlier, there was a 46 percent increase in AIDS cases reported in the primarily rural states in the South (Bell, 1991; the states included were Alabama, Georgia, Louisiana, Mississippi, North Carolina, South Carolina and Virginia). This same pattern has been seen nationwide; the National Commission on AIDS recently reported that the number of AIDS cases in rural communities increased 37 percent between early 1989 and early 1990 while the increase in cities of more than a half-million was only 5 percent.

The populations at risk of HIV infection have also changed with time, with adolescents at increasing risk. Even though reported cases of AIDS among persons 13 to 19 years of age account for only 0.4 percent of the cases in the United States, the total number of cases in this age group increased 25 percent during 1991 (Centers for Disease Control, 1992). As of December 1991, a total of 40,362 people between the ages of 20 and 29 had been diagnosed with AIDS in the United States (Centers for Disease Control, 1992). Given that a person can be infected with HIV for 10 years or more before symptoms of AIDS begin to develop, a significant number of those people were probably infected during adolescence.

In spite of national educational campaigns that have resulted in general awareness of HIV/AIDS and understanding of sexual transmission of HIV, adolescents continue to be involved in risky behaviors. Between 1986 and 1988, sexual activity among teenagers increased to the greatest proportional extent since 1970 (Centers for Disease Control, 1991). One recent survey of tenth grade students showed that by 15 years of age, 25 percent of the students reported engaging in activities that put them at high risk of acquiring HIV infection and 3 percent reported involvement in very high risk behavior (Walter, Vaughan and Cohall, 1991). There is growing concern that adolescents may be at substantial risk of HIV infection as a result of involvement in risk activities (DiClemente, 1990; Manoff et al., 1989). There is general agreement that, in the absence of a cure for AIDS, education about the risks of HIV exposure and infection is the most effective weapon in the fight against AIDS. A number of surveys and studies have shown that parents want their children to learn about AIDS and they want the schools to play a major role in that education. Almost all large school districts provide HIV/AIDS education to their students but smaller districts, characteristic of rural settings, are less likely to offer such education (General Accounting Office–Gap, 1990). The issues that teachers in larger school districts view as barriers to provision of HIV/AIDS and related sexuality education are probably more acute for rural teachers because of closer contact with school district patrons and smaller budgets. However, those barriers can be overcome.

Barriers

Rural school administrators almost unanimously endorse the need for and the value of HIV/AIDS education (Girvan and Salzman, 1990). Studies such as Kann et al. (1991) and Salzman and Girvan (1991) point out the critical nature of implementing a plan that helps young people acquire the knowledge and skills they need to adopt and maintain behaviors that reduce the risk of HIV infection. Many rural administrators report being directly involved in the planning and implementation of an AIDS prevention education curriculum in their district. However, they also note that few rural schools have structured programs in place

(Salzman and Girvan, 1991). From an administrative perspective, reasons for lack of a structured HIV/AIDS program generally relate to pressure or fear of pressure from parents and the community members or groups (Forrest and Silverman, 1989), a failure by the community and the student population to identify HIV and AIDS as "our problem" (Siegel and Gibson, 1988), a belief that knowledge will lead to irresponsible activity (University of Utah Health Behavior Laboratory, 1991), and lack of adoption of a policy which speaks to curricular issues.

Teachers, on the other hand, cite lack of administrative support, lack of funding for materials, inadequate knowledge and in-service training concerning how to teach about sensitive issues in the classroom, and lack of a defined, sequential, school board–approved curriculum as chief reasons for infrequent HIV/AIDS curricular implementation (Salzman & Girvan, 1991; AACD et al., 1990). In short, when teachers and administrators fail to take the time necessary to follow a deliberate curriculum development process, social issues like HIV and AIDS will continue to go unaddressed in the rural school setting. Students in rural areas practice risk behaviors in similar percentages to their counterparts in urban areas (Salzman & Girvan, 1991). The numbers of infected individuals have not reached the same levels in rural areas, so the potential for education to make an impact on this disease is far greater. In order to prevent further spread of HIV infection and protect young people, the aforementioned barriers must be overcome. Methods that have been used successfully to surmount the obstacles to implementation follow.

Implementation Procedure

As the primary purpose of health education is to promote adoption of behaviors that will support a healthy lifestyle (disease prevention) or to change behaviors that do not contribute to good health, HIV/AIDS education is of the utmost necessity. Because AIDS is a deadly disease, failure to integrate accurate information, decision-making activities, and skill building scenarios focused on reducing risk behaviors into the school curriculum has the potential to be life-threatening for students.

Successful HIV/AIDS prevention education programs have been developed in both urban and rural schools. Most certainly the majority of these successful program, regardless of the setting, were developed through a planned, sequential process, not a one-shot approach.

With development of any controversial curriculum, it is critical for the administrator or curriculum specialist to include a balanced input from a variety of school publics. As Luty (1988) states: "To do otherwise is to allow for parochial concerns of special interest groups to predominate." Balanced input can be achieved by

1. informing community groups, clubs and PTAs about the need for HIV/AIDS education,

2. involving parents on a district health advisory committee with teachers,

3. providing in-service training for the community regarding the issues associated with HIV and AIDS,

4. gathering support from community health professionals, and

5. emphasizing to all community patrons that the main purpose of the curriculum is to promote positive behaviors and save lives (Luty, 1988).

In other words, it must be stressed that the major reason the HIV/AIDS curriculum is being developed is because the community cares about its children. These initial steps are often easier to accomplish in a rural area than in an urban one because of the smaller numbers of people and the bonding and closeness associated with smaller communities. This is particularly true if the administrator makes certain to include people in "key" constituencies (those representative of local occupations, philosophies and religious organizations, and respected longtime community members) on the HIV/AIDS committee and if the administrator has resided for many years in that community and, therefore, is seen as an ally.

Studying the issues, educating the community, and facilitating input will also go a long way toward diminishing the "fear barrier" generated in administrators, teachers, and school boards because of vocal opposition groups. Growth comes with awareness (Luty, 1988).

Secondly, the advisory committee should

1. study recommendations relating to the proposed HIV/AIDS curriculum,

2. identify strengths and weaknesses of any related program currently being taught in the district,

3. recommend curricular actions in keeping with local values and needs, and

4. be available as an ongoing information resource to the community (Allensworth, 1991).

In addition, the advisory committee should help draft a policy statement that clearly articulates the goals and objectives of the district's HIV/AIDS curriculum. The policy should be specific as to what is taught in each grade level so teachers feel safe in knowing their parameters. Delineating the goals and objectives in an age-appropriate sequence also offers the benefit of program cohesiveness and allows for a smooth transition when personnel changes occur.

Once the curriculum is established, materials are selected. According to health teachers in many rural settings, lack of materials is a common problem.

Few rural districts possess individuals with the time and expertise to develop teaching materials. This problem is exacerbated at the primary level by the fact that almost no elementary teacher is a health specialist. Because of time constraints and because many teachers are not experts in all the HIV and AIDS-related topics they must cover, possibilities exist that inaccurate information or poorly written materials can be passed on to students (Girvan and Salzman, 1990). Having the advisory committee screen and choose from the many readily available materials on the market greatly diminishes both teacher workload and community bias and enhances the chances that a truly correlated instructional sequence will be utilized.

The final step prior to implementation involves the in-servicing of faculty, staff, and administrators. Even in school districts where formalized HIV/AIDS education is offered, teachers have often been expected to teach the program without adequate training (General Accounting Office–Teacher Training, 1990). Poor training is a major hindrance to program delivery. By providing in-service opportunities that focus not only on HIV/AIDS facts and information but also on decision-making models, methods to address sensitive issues, and examples of classroom skill building activities, district personnel will all be prepared to deliver and support an HIV/AIDS prevention education program that meets the needs of their community and their students (Girvan and Farrell, 1989). They will also better be able to break down the common stereotype that "AIDS is not our problem "by promoting the ideal that all persons living with AIDS (PLWAs) are human and worthy of care (Peters and Connell, 1990). Local ownership of the program is more important than any other factor in combatting the barriers to implementation.

Summary

The process described above is time consuming, but the benefits of community and school ownership and ease of implementation far outweigh the costs of shoddy, short-term solutions which actually foster opposition. Using the advisory committee process, many largely rural low-incidence states have gone from almost no school-based AIDS education programs to having nearly 50 percent of the districts implementing a program within a period of two to three years (Salzman and Girvan, 1991). Concerted efforts to continue this trend must be maintained. As rural communities pull together, the second disease "AFRAIDS" (acute fear relating to AIDS) begins to disappear, and HIV/AIDS curriculum implementation is seen as a source of pride and caring.

References

AACD, ASHA, NASN, NASP, NASW, and NASSNC (1990). "Guidelines for HIV and AIDS Student Support Services." *Journal of School Health,* 60:249–255.

Allensworth, D. (1987). "Building Community Support for Quality School Health Programs." *Health Education,* 18:32–38.

Bell, N. K. (1991). "Social/Sexual Norms and AIDS in the South." *AIDS Education and Prevention,* 3:164–180.

Centers for Disease Control (1981). "Pneumocystis Pneumonia—Los Angeles." *Morbidity and Mortality Weekly Report,* 30:250–252.

____ (1991). "Premarital Sexual Experience Among Adolescent Women." *Morbidity and Mortality Weekly* Report, 39:929–932.

____ (1992, January). *HIV/AIDS Surveillance Report,* pp. 6, 13.

DiClemente, R. J. (1990). "The Emergence of Adolescents as a Risk Group for Human Immunodeficiency Virus Infection." *Journal of Adolescent Research,* 5:5–17.

Forrest, J. D., and Silverman, J. (1989). "What Public School Teachers Teach About Preventing Pregnancy, AIDS and Sexually Transmitted Diseases." *Family Planning Perspectives,* 21:56–64.

Girvan, J. T., and Farrell, L. D. (1989). "Developing an Effective Half-Day Secondary School Inservice on AIDS." *The Clearing House,* 62:381–383.

____ and Salzman, S. A. (1990). *Final Report: Assessment of Idaho HIV/AIDS Prevention Education Programs.* Boise: Idaho Department of Education.

Kann, L.; Anderson, J.; Holtzman, D.; Ross, J.; Truman, B. I.; Collins, J.; and Kolbe, L. J. (1991). "HIV-Related Knowledge, Beliefs and Behaviors Among High School Students in the United States: Results from a National Survey." *Journal of School Health,* 61:397–401.

Luty, E. T. (1988). "Controversial Topics in a Health Curriculum Program." *Health Education,* 5:39–44.

Manoff, S. B.; Gayle, H. D.; Mays, M. A.; and Rogers, M. F. (1989). "Acquired Immunodeficiency Syndrome in Adolescents: Epidemiology, Prevention and Public Health Issues." *Pediatric Infectious Diseases,* 8:309–314.

Oetter, D. (1987). "Comprehensive School Health Education: Overcoming Barriers." *Health Education,* 18:39–40.

Peters, F. L., and Connell, K. M. (1991). "Incorporating the Affective Component Into an AIDS Workshop." *Journal of Continuing Education in Nursing,* 22:95–99.

Salzman, S. A., and Girvan, J. T. (1991). "Evaluation of AIDS Prevention Education Programs: A Rural Schools Model." ERIC document no. TMO16243.

Siegel, K., and Gibson, W. C. (1988). "Barriers to the Modification of Sexual Behavior Among Heterosexuals at Risk for Acquired Immunodeficiency Syndrome." *New York State Journal of Medicine,* 88:66–70.

Silverman, M. F. (1990, January). "AIDS Crossroads: Fighting Burnout as Needs Swell." *The Nation's Health,* p. 24.

Stout, H. (1987, November 29). "40% of Americans Fear They Will Contract AIDS, a Poll Indicates." *The New York Times,* p. 26.

U.S. General Accounting Office (1990). "AIDS Education: Gaps in Coverage Still Exist." Testimony before the Senate Committee on Governmental Affairs. Washington, DC.

____ (1990). "AIDS Education: Public School Programs Require More Student Information and Teacher Training." Washington, DC.

University of Utah Health Behavior Laboratory (1991). *1991 Idaho Youth Risk Behavior and School Health Education Survey Report.* November.

Walter, H. J.; Vaughan, R. D.; and Cohall, A. T. (1991). "Psychosocial Influences on Acquired Immunodeficiency Syndrome–Risk Behaviors Among High School Students." *Pediatrics,* 88:846–852.

Chapter Seven

The Status of AIDS/HIV Education in the Professional Preparation of Preservice Elementary Teachers

DAVID M. WHITE
DANNY J. BALLARD

As this manuscript was being prepared during the 1992 AIDS Conference in Stockholm, Sweden, the consensus opinion of the experts at this meeting was that prevention, through education, remains the best way to fight this deadly disease. Supporters of school-based AIDS/HIV education point out that elementary and secondary schools can educate up to 95 percent of youth about HIV infection (Black & Jones, 1988). Objective number 18.10 of *Healthy People 2000: National Health Promotion and Disease Promotion Objectives* (U.S. Department of Health and Human Services, 1990) seeks to "increase to at least 95 percent the proportion of schools that have age-appropriate HIV education curricula for students in 4th through 12th grade, preferably as a part of quality school health education." Authorities and organizations have recommended that schools have in-service programs to prepare teachers to provide AIDS education (Centers for Disease Control, 1988; Reinzo & Dorman, 1988; Watkins, 1988; Strouse and Phillips, 1987). Kerr, Allensworth, and Gayle (1989) documented the significant need for training teachers about HIV/AIDS issues. This need should be addressed not only through in-service training, but also within the preservice component of the professional education curriculum.

This article, the research for which was funded through a grant from the Texas A&M College of Education, is reprinted with permission from the Journal of Health Education, *March/April 1993, 24(2): 68–72.* Journal of Health Education *is a publication of the American Alliance for Health, Physical Education, Recreation and Dance, 1900 Association Drive, Reston, Virginia 22091.*

The Centers for Disease Control (CDC) (1989) have recommended that colleges of education assure provision of preservice instruction about AIDS.

Providing adequate instruction about AIDS within professional education programs for elementary teachers appears to be a challenge. We reviewed the course requirements for elementary education majors at several universities. This informal view revealed that the typical elementary education major receives AIDS/HIV instruction in no more than one course, and this most likely is in a health education class. The elementary education major may be receiving very little preservice education about AIDS and HIV, yet he or she is expected to address AIDS-related issues competently and professionally in the elementary school classroom. Ballard, White, and Glascoff (1990) surveyed elementary education majors and found general agreement that they would eventually have a child with AIDS in the classroom and that AIDS education should be taught in the elementary grades. However, more than one-fifth of the sample did not believe they understood the basics about AIDS. Only one-half stated they could comfortably answer elementary students' questions about AIDS. Fewer than one-half said they knew how to protect themselves from HIV in the classroom, and less than one-third said they knew how to clean up blood or body fluids safely. A survey of preservice education majors about AIDS (Cinelli, Sandaran, McConatha, & Carson, 1992) revealed misconceptions about HIV transmission and HIV antibody testing and policies and procedures related to AIDS, such as knowing that the parents of children in school have no right to information regarding the HIV status of other children in the school. The evidence points to a need to examine the status of AIDS/HIV instruction as a component of the preservice training of elementary school teachers.

The purpose of this chapter was to conduct a nationwide survey of professional education programs to determine the preparation of preservice elementary teachers to teach about AIDS and HIV and to manage issues related to the disease in the classroom.

Method

Sample The sample comprised all colleges and universities listed in the 1990 directory of the American Association of Colleges in Teacher Education (AACTE). This listing was considered to be the most comprehensive one available for the purpose of conducting a national survey of institutions with professional education programs. Approximately 700 institutions were listed in the directory, and 197 completed surveys were received for a 28 percent return rate.

Survey Instrument No suitable instrument could be found that addressed the project's purpose; therefore the survey tool was developed by the writers. A series of open-ended and closed-ended items were constructed to respond to the project's objectives. These items and a list of the project objectives were reviewed by two education school deans, three elementary school teachers, four health education professors, and four elementary education professors. Revisions were based on their suggestions. The final form of the instrument includes 10 closed-ended items and 10 open-ended items. Several items focus on the planned instruction within elementary education curricula about (a) the cause, transmission, and prevention of AIDS, (b) providing AIDS education (how to teach about AIDS), and (c) dealing with the possibility that a child with AIDS or HIV might be in the classroom. These items are separated according to grade-level emphasis, being grouped as targeting either primary grades, defined as grades K–3, or intermediate and middle grades, defined as grades 4–6. Other items ask about the course(s) that elementary education majors take that have planned instruction about AIDS and HIV—specifically, which academic units provide the courses and whether or not they are required courses for elementary majors. Finally, items about resources used and needed for AIDS/HIV instruction are included.

Procedure The revised survey instrument was mailed to all institutions listed in the 1990 edition of the AACTE directory. Generally, the questionnaires were addressed to either the dean or the director of the college or school of education, or to the chair of the elementary education unit, depending on the way the unit was listed in the directory. There were two mailings. The first was sent out in spring 1990. The follow-up mailing was sent out during the summer of 1990 to those who did not respond to the first mailing.

Results

Instruction About the Cause, Transmission, and Prevention of AIDS The first series of items focused on the instruction that elementary education majors with a primary grades (K–3) emphasis receive about the cause, transmission, and prevention of AIDS. The first item asked if elementary education majors with an emphasis on primary grades received planned instruction about the cause, transmission, and prevention of AIDS. Of the 193 respondents who answered this item, 106 (54.9 percent) said "yes," 78 (40.4 percent) said "no," and 9 (4.7 percent) said "I don't know." Those who answered "yes" were asked to estimate the amount of class time (in minutes) and the number of class periods spent on this topic. There were 102 respondents to this item. The mean amount of class time given was 99.5 minutes, with a range of 10 to 300 minutes. The standard deviation of the responses was 53.0 minutes and the mode was 60 minutes. The number of class periods ranged from one to six, with an average of 1.8 and standard deviation of 1.0. The mode was one class period.

The next item asked if elementary majors with a middle or intermediate grades emphasis (4–6) received planned instruction about the cause, transmission, and prevention of AIDS. Of the 191 respondents to this item, 111 (58.1

percent) said "yes," 73 (38.2 percent) said "no," and 7 (3.7 percent) said "I don't know." Of the 111 respondents who said "yes," 108 answered the question about amount of class time and number of class periods spent on this topic. The average was 108 minutes, with a range of 10 to 300 minutes. The standard deviation of responses was 98.8 minutes and the mode was 60 minutes. The average number of class periods devoted to this topic was 1.8, with a range of one to six class periods. The standard deviation of responses was 1.0 and the mode was one class period.

An open-ended item asked what information was included in this planned instruction about the cause, transmission and prevention of AIDS for elementary education majors. Most respondents answered that instruction included information concerning the causes, means of transmission, and ways to prevent AIDS. Others indicated that this instruction included discussion of general information, such as current status, projected status, clarifying myths, symptoms, ways to avoid risky behaviors (assertiveness and communication skills), social implications, effects (physical and mental), student concerns, and persons with AIDS or HIV in the class. Some respondents stated that this was accomplished by presenting teaching techniques and requiring students to develop lesson plans for teaching the subject; having guest speakers, videos, and handouts; obtaining information from the CDC and Red Cross; and knowing state and local school policies. Implementing AIDS instruction within STD instruction was also a common response, along with teaching about abstinence, monogamy, condoms, homophobia, and human sexuality.

These items were followed by a question that asked what courses elementary education majors take that include planned instruction about the cause, transmission, and prevention of AIDS. The respondents listed the course number and name, and indicated whether or not it was a required course. We examined the course prefixes to determine in which academic unit the course was offered. The academic unit mentioned most frequently was health education, with 112 (65 percent) of the courses listed. Of these, 96 were required courses and 16 were not required. Thirty-seven (21 percent) of the courses listed had a prefix which indicated that they were taught in the education department. Thirty-two of these courses were required and five were not required. The remaining 23 (13.5 percent) courses listed were found in the psychology unit, the physical education unit, and other specified units. Of the 162 courses listed, 140 (86.4 percent) were required and 22 (13.6 percent) were not required.

Instruction About Providing AIDS/HIV Education The next series of items focused on the planned instruction that elementary education majors receive about providing age appropriate AIDS/HIV education (how to teach about AIDS and HIV). First, respondents were asked if elementary education majors with a primary grades emphasis receive this type of instruction. Of the 189 responses, 68 (36.2 percent) said "yes," 104 (55.3 percent) said "no," and 16 (8.5 percent) said "I don't know." Of the 68 respondents who said "yes," 66 answered the questions about class time and number of class periods spent on this topic. The average estimated amount of class time was 77.9 minutes, with a range of 15 to 300 minutes. The standard deviation was 57.9 minutes and the mode was 30 minutes. The average number of class periods was 1.5, with a range of one to six periods. The standard deviation was 1.0 and the mode was one class period.

The next item asked if elementary education majors with a middle or intermediate grades emphasis receive planned instruction about providing age-appropriate AIDS/HIV education for students in the intermediate and middle grades. Of the 188 respondents, 72 (38.3 percent) said "yes," 101 (53.7 percent) said "no," and 15 (8.0 percent) said "I don't know." Seventy of the 72 who answered "yes" responded to the items asking about class time and number of class periods devoted to this topic. The average number of minutes indicated was 78.1, with a range of 15 to 300 minutes. The standard deviation was 56.1 minutes and the mode was 60 minutes. The average number of class periods indicated was 1.7, with a range of one to nine class periods. The standard deviation of responses was 1.3 and the mode was one class period.

An open-ended item followed that asked what information elementary majors with a primary grades emphasis receive pertaining to planned instruction about providing age-appropriate AIDS/HIV education for elementary school students. Forty-seven respondents answered this item. Nineteen (40.4 percent) stated they taught strategies or methodologies in AIDS education; 10 (21.3 percent) used state and local curriculum guidelines; 8 (17 percent) taught cause, transmission, and prevention of AIDS; and the remaining 10 (21.3 percent) included AIDS curricula from sources such as the Red Cross, and accompanied this with classroom handouts, activities, and lectures on human sexuality.

A total of 89 courses were listed in response to the question "What courses do elementary education majors take that include planned instruction about providing age-appropriate AIDS/HIV education?" Sixty-one (68.5 percent) were offered by the health education unit, 53 were required courses and 8 were not required. The education unit was indicated for 25 courses, with 24 required and 1 not required. The remaining 2 (3.5 percent) were from the psychology unit and the physical education unit. Both were required courses. In all, 80 of the courses were listed as required and 8 were not required.

Instruction About Dealing with a Child with AIDS or HIV The next items asked whether elementary education majors receive planned instruction about dealing with a child with AIDS or HIV infection in the classroom. Of the 189 respondents, 88 (46.6 percent) said "yes," 82 (43.4 percent) said "no," and 19 (10.1 percent) said "I don't know." Eighty-three of the 88 respondents who said "yes" responded to items asking about amount of class time and number of class periods devoted to this topic. The average amount of class time indicated was 56.5 minutes, with a range of 10 to 200 minutes. The standard deviation was 43.2 minutes and the mode was 30 minutes. The average number of class periods indicated was 1.4, with a range of one to nine periods. The standard deviation was 1.1, and the mode was one class period.

The next item asked if elementary education majors with a middle or intermediate grades emphasis received planned instruction about dealing with the possibility that a child with AIDS or HIV infection might be in the classroom. Of the 186 respondents, 89 (47.8 percent) said "yes," 79 (42.5 percent) said "no," and 18 (9.7 percent) said "I don't know." Eighty-four of the 89 who said "yes" answered the items about amount of class time and number of class periods spent on this topic. The mean amount of time was 54.7 minutes, with a range of 10 to 200 minutes. The standard deviation of responses was 40.9 minutes and the mode was 60 minutes. The average number of class periods spent on this topic was 1.3, with a range of one to nine class periods. The standard deviation was 1.1 periods, and the mode was one period.

There was a total of 60 responses to the open-ended part of this item that asked what is included in the instruction received by elementary education majors about dealing with the possibility that a child with AIDS or HIV infection might be in the classroom. Seventeen responses (28.3 percent) dealt primarily with confidentiality, safe handling of blood and body fluids, and helping other students understand their classmate with AIDS/HIV; 14 (23.3 percent) stressed the cause, transmission and prevention of AIDS; 10 (6.0 percent) said instruction was centered around state and local policies; and the remaining 19 (42.4 percent) respondents said the planned instruction concentrated on a wide variety of AIDS/HIV and health-related areas. There were 92 courses listed in response to the question asking about courses that elementary education majors take which include planned instruction about dealing with a child with AIDS or HIV infection. Forty-four (47.8 percent) were offered by the health education unit; 43 were required courses and 1 was not a required course. Thirty-three (35.9 percent) courses were offered by the education unit; 32 were listed as required courses and 1 was not required. The remaining 14 (15.2 percent) were from the psychology unit, the physical education unit, and other unspecified unit; 13 were required courses, and 1 was not required.

Resources The final items on the questionnaire were open-ended questions that asked about resources used when teaching elementary education majors about AIDS. A wide variety of responses were received. The most common sources of information were state curriculum guidelines, Centers for Disease Control publications, American Red Cross materials, and public health department information. Guest speakers listed frequently were physicians, community health educators, AIDS counselors, and school nurses. A variety of books and videotapes were indicated as resources for instruction. Respondents were asked to suggest additional resources and teaching aids that would be helpful. Again, a variety of responses were given. Several respondents indicated that there was not enough time in the curriculum to cover the topic adequately.

Some said that they were "not as far along as we should be," and they often requested a curriculum developed specifically for elementary education majors. Several respondents suggested that videotapes be made available that included interviews with elementary teachers who have dealt with children with AIDS and interviews of parents of elementary children with AIDS. Filmed sessions of model teachers instructing children about AIDS and demonstrating teaching strategies to use in elementary classrooms were also requested.

Conclusions

Results of this national survey indicate that a substantial percentage of professional preparation programs do not include instruction about AIDS and HIV for preservice elementary teachers. Just over half the programs surveyed include planned instruction about the cause, transmission, and prevention of AIDS and HIV for elementary education majors. Less than half of these programs include instruction on teaching about AIDS and HIV and dealing with the possibility that a child with AIDS or HIV infection may be in the classroom. There is clearly a large gap between what is recommended by disease prevention authorities and what is actually taking place in the professional preparation programs. There did seem to be a recognition of the need for this type of instruction among the administrators of professional education programs. The major constraint listed was finding time within the curriculum to provide this instruction. The health education unit was generally the source of courses for providing this instruction; however, the amount of time spent on AIDS education was limited, generally only one class period. The respondents indicated that they did use a wide variety of AIDS educational resources. They also made suggestions for additional resources.

Recommendations

Results of this survey indicate that professional preparation programs do not, as a rule, include planned instruction about AIDS for elementary education majors. Those that do typically look to the health education unit for instruction about AIDS. Health education faculty should work with elementary education faculty to determine appropriate guidelines for developing and evaluating the AIDS/HIV educational component of the teacher preparation programs. Health educators should address the need for including appropriate AIDS/HIV education in professional preparation programs through elementary education professional societies and their journals. Several excellent suggestions were made about development of videotapes and other instructional aids. A problem noted by many respondents was a lack of time for this instruction. Elementary education faculty and administrators should carefully review their priorities for preparation of elementary teachers. Education in HIV and AIDS, particularly within the framework of comprehensive school health education, is of critical importance and should maintain a high position in these priorities. Future research should investigate other professional education disciplines, such as science education and home economics education, because these areas are also expected to include instruction in the public schools about AIDS and HIV. Since the main avenue for halting the spread of this deadly disease is through education, professional education programs should address the need to prepare preservice elementary teachers to teach about AIDS and HIV and to manage issues related to AIDS and HIV in the classroom.

References

Ballard, D.; White, D.; and Glascoff, M. (1990). "AIDS/HIV Education for Preservice Elementary Teachers." *Journal of School Health,* 60(6):262–265.

Black, J., and Jones, L. (1988). "HIV Infection: Educational Programs and Policies for School Personnel." *Journal of School Health,* 58(8):317–321.

Cinelli, B.; Sankaran, G.; McConatha, D.; and Carsoll, L. (1992). "Knowledge and Attitudes of Pre-Service Education Majors About AIDS: Implications for Curriculum Development." *Journal of Health Education,* 23(4):204–208.

Kerr, D.; Allensworth, D.; and Gayle, J. (1989). "The ASHA National HIV Education Needs Assessment of Health and Education Professionals." *Journal of School Health,* 59(7):301–307.

Reinzo, B., and Dorman, S. (1988). "Ten Consequences of the AIDS Crisis for the Health Education Profession." *Journal of School Health,* 58(8):335–338.

Strouse, J., and Phillips, J. (1987). "Teaching About AIDS: A Challenge to Educators." *Educational Leader,* 44(7):76–80.

U.S. Department of Health and Human Services (1990). *Healthy People 2000: National Health Promotion and Disease Prevention Objectives.* Washington, DC: U.S. Government Printing Office.

Watkins, J. (1988). *Report of the Presidential Commission on the Human Immunodeficiency Virus Epidemic.* Washington, DC: Presidential Commission on the Human Immunodeficiency Virus Epidemic. U.S. Government Printing Office, publication no. 0-214-701.

Chapter Eight

AIDS in the Classroom: Are Teacher Attitudes Changing?

BENJAMIN W. BRUCKER
WAYNE H. HALL

In 1987 a survey was administered to a group of teachers attending graduate school at Eastern Washington University in Cheney, Washington. The survey asked teachers a variety of questions on issues related to Acquired Immune Deficiency Syndrome (AIDS). Results of the survey indicated that the teachers were divided on many of these issues. Teachers, in general, had not given much thought to such questions as whether all teachers should be required to teach children infected with the AIDS virus or whether mandatory AIDS testing of teachers should be required for certification.

Since the original survey was conducted in 1987, the general public, including teachers, has become more educated and knowledgeable on AIDS-related issues. Numerous television programs have been broadcast nationally in an attempt to educate society on how AIDS is and is not transmitted, who is at risk, and many issues related to the fear of AIDS. The media has launched an aggressive campaign to educate the public about AIDS in an attempt to alleviate many of myths and fears concerning AIDS. The majority of school districts in the country have now adopted parent and school board approved AIDS curriculums. In many of the schools, these programs begin as early as third grade. Additionally, numerous teachers have been trained or have been required to attend at least one in-service session on AIDS. Many states now include an AIDS curriculum as part of teacher training programs.

When the first survey was administered in 1987, the Associated Press reported that the Centers for Disease Control (CDC) stated that the majority of AIDS cases came from homosexual activity and intravenous drug use. Now,

CDC reports that these figures are changing and AIDS is spreading to the heterosexual community. Thus, society is beginning to realize that AIDS is anyone's disease; it is a disease that could possibly infect anyone from any segment of society.

Generally speaking, teachers now have more information than in 1987 on which to base personal decisions regarding AIDS issues. As a result, the hysteria and fear that abounded when the original study was conducted should have abated somewhat. In an effort to test this assumption, a survey was administered during the summer of 1991 to approximately 400 students attending summer session at Eastern Washington University. The survey consisted of the same 13 statements used in the 1987 survey; respondents indicated whether they strongly agreed, agreed, disagreed, strongly disagreed, or had no opinion on each statement. The age of the respondents completing the survey ranged from 23 years to 62 years. The majority of students (73 percent) were in the 26 to 45 year age range. Of the respondents, 87 were male and 256 were female. Eight states were represented in the survey including Washington, Idaho, California, Oregon, Montana, and Colorado, with 326 of the respondents from the state of Washington. Most teachers in the survey had less than ten years of teaching experience. Respondents completing the survey were from communities ranging from fewer than 1,000 people to communities with populations over 250,000, with the majority coming from communities with populations under 100,000. Also, teachers completing the survey represented grades from K to 12 with the majority of teachers in the K to 6 range.

This chapter attempts to determine whether teacher attitudes toward AIDS changed during the period between the 1987 and 1991 surveys.

Data Analysis

The analyses of the data consisted of two distinct components:

A. An analysis to attempt to determine if the percentage of responses to each of the 13 items had changed from the responses of 1987.

B. Four different analyses to determine if different groupings of respondents responded to each of the items in a different way. The groupings of respondents consisted of:

1. *Age Levels:* Under 25, 26–35, 36–45, 46–55.
2. *Sex:* Males, Females
3. *Grades Taught During Major Part of Day:* K–3, 4–6, 7–9, 10–12, Other.
4. *Highest Degree Earned:* Bachelor's Degree, 5th Year/Certification Level, Master's Degree.

The results of the analyses will be addressed in two corresponding sections.

Section A. The purpose of this component of the analysis was to attempt to determine if the attitudes of teachers towards AIDS changed in the time between the two surveys. For each of the 13 items, the categories of Strongly Agree and Agree were combined. For each of these combined categories, and the No Opinion category, a proportions test was administered to determine whether the percent of responses to each item had changed in the period since the first survey. Each of the analyses was conducted at the .05 level of significance. The percentage of responses for each category along with the percentage of combined responses for Strongly Agree and Agree are presented in Table 8.1 for both summer 1991 and summer 1987.

It can be seen from the information provided in Table 8.1 that the percent of respondents having no opinion was extremely small in both 1987 and 1991, and the analyses indicate that the percent of responses to the No Opinion category did not change significantly for any of the items. However, in the combined categories of Strongly Agree and Agree, it can be seen that there was a significant change in the percentage response for 12 of the 13 items. The only item in which there was not a significant change from the summer of 1987 to the summer of 1991 was item 12 ("Teachers should be required to teach students infected with AIDS only if the students display 'no outward signs' ").

Of the 12 items in which a significant change occurred, several of the items stand out. For example, item 2 ("All beginning teachers should be required to be tested for the AIDS antibody as a requirement for certification") had a 45 percent combined response (SA+A) in 1987 and a 25.4 percent response in 1991. Item 3 ("If a teacher tests positive for the AIDS virus, he or she should not be allowed to teach") had a 46 percent combined response (SA+A) in 1987 and only a 17.8 percent response in 1991. Thirty-one percent of the teachers surveyed either strongly agreed or agreed with item 6 ("Students who have been infected with the AIDS virus should not be allowed to attend classes") in 1987 whereas in the 1991 survey only 8.9 percent strongly agreed or agreed. In item 7 ("Students who have been infected with the AIDS virus should not be allowed to participate in school activities with other students"), 34 percent of the teachers had a combined response (SA+A) in 1987 and a 19.9 percent combined response (SA+A) in 1991.

The analyses of these other 12 items indicate that the summer of 1991 teachers are less negative toward the issues related to AIDS than the summer 1987 teachers in every case.

Section B. This component of the analysis consisted of attempting to determine if different groupings responded to each of the items in a different way. This consisted of an analysis of each of the 13 items for each of four different groupings. Each of the analyses was conducted at the .05 level of significance. The results are as follows:

1. Age Levels: Under 25, 26–35, 36–45, 46–55. A simple one-way analysis of variance (ANOVA) was conducted for each of the 13 questions in an

Table 8.1: Attitudes to AIDS in the Classroom

Question	*SA*	*A*	*Response* *D*	*SD*	*NO*	*Combined Response SA&A*
1. All teachers should be required to be tested for AIDS.	17% 8.7	30% 24.6	30% 39.0	19% 21.8	4% 5.6	47%★ 33.3★★
2. All beginning teachers should be required to be tested for the AIDS antibody as a requirement for certification.	19% 7.6	26% 17.8	30% 42.6	23% 28.4	2% 3.4	45% 25.4
3. If a teacher tests positive for the AIDS virus, he or she should not be allowed to teach.	20% 4.5	26% 13.3	29% 52.1	18% 24.9	7% 5.0	46% 17.8
4. If a teacher's test indicates that he or she has been infected with the AIDS virus but shows "no outward signs," he or she should be issued a teaching certificate.	13% 17.6	45% 53.1	23% 16.4	15% 5.9	4% 6.8	58% 70.7
5. Mandatory testing of students (K–12) for the AIDS antibody should be required for all students as a condition for his or her attending class.	10% 3.9	16% 14.4	41% 45.1	27% 32.1	6% 4.2	26% 18.3
6. Students (K–12) who have been infected with the AIDS virus should not be allowed to attend classes.	15% 1.9	16% 7.0	41% 43.3	23% 43.6	5% 3.9	31% 8.9
7. Students (K–12) who have been infected with the AIDS virus should not be allowed to participate in school activities with other students.	13% 12.8	21% 7.1	40% 44.7	21% 41.0	6% 4.2	34% 19.9
8. Students (K–12) who have been infected with the AIDS virus but who display "no outward signs" should be allowed to attend classes.	18% 27.5	42% 55.9	23% 9.6	12% 2.5	5% 4.2	60% 83.4
9. Students (K–12) who have been infected with the AIDS virus but who display "no outward signs" should be allowed to participate in school activities with other students.	15% 26.3	45% 64.4	22% 11.1	12% 3.4	6% 4.5	60% 80.7

Table 8.1: Continued.

Question	*SA*	*A*	*Response* *D*	*SD*	*NO*	*Combined Response SA&A*
10. School districts should take appropriate steps to educate students, parents and school employees regarding AIDS and its transmission.	76% 80.7	14% 16.7	5% .8	4% .8	1% .8	90% 97.4
11. Teachers (K–12) should not be required to teach students infected with AIDS.	14% 6.8	22% 13.3	34% 42.4	24% 31.9	6% 6.4	36% 20.1
12. Teachers (K–12) should be required to teach students infected with AIDS only if the students display "no outward signs."	8% 9.1	28% 27.1	32% 35.7	24% 18.8	8% 9.1	36% 36.2
13. Public school districts have a responsibility to provide an educational program for those who are infected with the AIDS virus.	37% 51.6	38% 37.5	9% 5.9	10% 1.6	6% 3.1	75% 89.1

SA=Strongly Agree; A=Agree; D=Disagree; SD=Strongly Disagree; NO=No opinion
SA%+A%=Total # of Strongly Agree and Agree Responses
Significant at the .05 level*
★=Answers given in 1987 poll. ★★=Answers given in 1991 poll.

attempt to determine if there was any difference in the responses among the different age levels. Of the 13 items analyzed, a significant overall F was found for only one item. This item was item 11 ("Teachers [K–12] should not be required to teach students infected with AIDS"). The results of the overall ANOVA for item 11 is provided in Table 8.2.

The mean, standard deviation and sample size for each group are presented in Table 8.3. An analysis of the means of the groups indicates that the age group of 36–45 had a significantly different average response to item 11 than either the under 25 age group or the 26–35 age group. Since the Strongly Agree response is scaled at 4 and the average response ranges from 1.72 to 2.04, it is evident that, overall, the teachers tended to disagree with this item. However, this result indicates that the 36–45 age group of teachers tended to agree more strongly than either of two other age groups that teachers should not be required to teach students with AIDS.

2. Sex: Males, Females. A t-test was conducted for each of the 13 items to attempt to determine if there was a difference in the responses to items rela-

**Represents the probability of the measured association being due to sampling error.*

Table 8.2: Age-Related Variance Analysis: Item 11

Source of Variation	*Sums of Squares*	*Degrees of Freedom*	*Mean Squares*	*Test Statistics*
Treatments	7.70	3	2.57	2.83
Experimental Error	313.34	346	0.91	
Total	321.04	349		

Significant at .05 level.

Table 8.3: Age-Related Mean and Standard Deviation: Item 11

	Under 25	*26–35*	*36–45*	*46–55*
Mean	1.73	1.72	2.04	1.85
ST.D.	.93	.93	.93	1.20
N	67	138	118	27

tive to the sex of the individuals. In the 13 analyses conducted, a significant difference was found for only three of the items. The mean, standard deviation and sample size for each of the items are provided in Table 8.4.

The first of the items in which a difference was found was item 3 ("If a teacher tests positive for the AIDS virus, he or she should not be allowed to teach"). Although both males and females tended to disagree with this item, the males disagreed less strongly than the females. This indicates that the males were more likely than the females to agree that a teacher who tests positive for the AIDS virus should not be allowed to teach.

The second item in which a significant difference was found was item 6 ("Students who have been infected with the AIDS virus should not be allowed to attend classes"). Again, both males and females tended to disagree with this item, but again the males disagreed less strongly than the females. This also indicates that the males were more likely than the females to agree that students who have AIDS should not be allowed to attend classes.

The third item in which a significant difference was found was item 8 ("Students who have been infected with the AIDS virus but display 'no outward signs' should be allowed to attend classes"). This was an item with which both males and females tended to agree. However, the males tended to agree less strongly than the females, again indicating that males have a stronger negative attitude towards this issue than the females.

The results of these analyses indicate that the males have a more negative attitude towards the issues addressed by all three of these items.

3. Grades Taught During Major Part of Day: K–3, 4–6, 7–9, 10–12, K–12, other. An ANOVA was conducted for each of the 13 questions to attempt

Table 8.4: Gender-Related Mean and Standard Deviation

	Males	*Females*
Item 3		
Mean	2.14	1.90
ST.D.	.87	.73
N	83	239
t=2.26#		
Item 6		
Mean	1.82	1.60
ST.D.	.83	.66
N	83	243
t=2.14#		
Item 8		
Mean	2.98	3.17
ST.D.	.79	.66
N	82	242
t=2.05#		

Significant at the .05 level

to determine if there were differences in responses among the different levels of grades taught. Of the thirteen items analyzed, there were three items to which a significantly different response was found based on the grade level at which the teachers were teaching. One of the items in which there was a significant difference is item 4 ("If a teacher's test indicates that he or she has been infected with the AIDS virus but shows 'no outward signs,' he or she should be issued a teaching certificate"). The results of the overall ANOVA for item 4 are provided in Table 8.5.

Table 8.5: Grade Level Variance Analysis: Item 4

Source of Variation	*SS*	*DF*	*MS*	*F*
Treatments	14.06	5	2.81	2.63#
Experimental Error	322.36	302	1.07	
Total	336.43	307		

Significant at .05 level.

Table 8.6: Grade Level Mean and Standard Deviation: Item 4

Grades	*K–3*	*4–6*	*7–9*	*10–12*	*K–12*	*Other*
Mean	2.81	2.77	2.70	2.55	2.15	2.31
ST.D.	.87	.97	1.23	1.27	1.27	1.32
N	108	53	44	41	20	42

The mean, standard deviation and sample size for each group are provided in Table 8.6. Overall, the teachers tended to agree slightly with this statement.However, the teachers in kindergarten through sixth grade were significantly more positive in their response than the K–12 teachers and those in the "Other" category. Also, the teachers in the K–12 group were significantly less positive to this item than the 7–9 grade group.

The second item for which there was a significant disagreement among the responses was item 7 ("Students [K–12] who have been infected with the AIDS virus should not be allowed to participate in school activities with other students"). The results of the overall ANOVA for item 7 are presented in Table 8.7.

Table 8.7: Grade Level Analysis of Variance: Item 7

Source of Variation	*SS*	*DF*	*MS*	*F*
Treatments	9.25	5	1.85	2.88#
Experimental Error	193.20	301	0.64	
Total	202.44	306		

Significant at .05 level.

The mean, standard deviation and sample size for each of the groups are provided in Table 8.8. The concept that K–12 students who have been infected with the AIDS virus should not be allowed to participate in school activities with other students was disagreed with fairly strongly by the teachers at all grade levels. However, the K–12 group of teachers disagreed more strongly than the teachers at the K–3 level, the teachers at the 7–9 level and the teachers at the 10–12 level. Also, the teachers at the 7–9 level did not disagree as strongly as the teachers at the 4–6 level and the "Other" grade level teachers.

The third item for which there was a significant difference among the responses was item 11 ("Teachers [K–12] should not be required to teach students infected with AIDS"). The results of the overall ANOVA are presented in Table 8.9.

Table 8.8: Grade Level Mean and Standard Deviation: Item 7

Grades	*K–3*	*4–6*	*7–9*	*10–12*	*K–12*	*Other*
Mean	1.70	1.56	1.89	1.83	1.19	1.55
ST.D.	.78	.75	.72	.96	.81	.83
N	108	52	44	40	21	42

Table 8.9: Grade Level Analysis of Variance: Item 11

Source of Variation	*SS*	*DF*	*MS*	*F*
Treatments	10.45	5	2.09	2.28#
Experimental Error	276.56	301	0.92	
Total	287.0	306		

Significant at .05 level.

Table 8.10: Grade Level Mean and Standard Deivation: Item 11

Grades	*K–3*	*4–6*	*7–9*	*10–12*	*K–12*	*Other*
Mean	1.97	1.89	2.14	1.90	1.57	1.55
ST.D.	.96	.89	1.04	1.00	.98	.92
N	107	53	43	41	21	42

The mean, standard deviation and sample size for each of the groups are provided in Table 8.10. This was an item with which there was relatively strong disagreement among all of the teachers. However, those teachers at the 7–9 grade level did not disagree as strongly with this item as did the teachers at the K–12 level and those teaching at the "Other" grade level.

4. Highest Degree Earned: Bachelor's Degree, 5th Level, Master's Degree. An ANOVA was conducted for each of the 13 questions in an attempt to determine if there was any difference in the responses among the three levels of degrees earned. Of the 13 items analyzed, a significant overall F was found for only one item, namely item 11 ("Teachers [K–12] should not be required to teach students infected with AIDS"). The results of the overall ANOVA for item 11 are presented in Table 8.11.

The mean, standard deviation and sample size for each of the groups are

Table 8.11: Degrees Earned Analysis of Variance: Item 11

Source of Variation	*SS*	*DF*	*MS*	*F*
Treatments	5.61	2	2.80	3.14#
Experimental Error	272.81	305	0.89	
Total	277.79	307		

Significant at .05 level.

Table 8.12: Degree Earned Standard Deviation: Item 11

	Bachelor's	*5th Yr. Cert.*	*Master's*
Mean	1.82	1.85	2.26
ST.D.	.95	.86	1.19
N	154	120	34

provided in Table 8.12. An analysis of the means of the groups indicates that the teachers who had completed their master's degree responded differently to this item from either of the other two groups. The master's degree group tended to be more likely to agree that teachers should not be required to teach students with AIDS.

Discussions, Conclusions, Summary

In 1991 the teachers, in general, seemed to feel less threatened by the whole issue of AIDS and less negative toward those with the disease. In 1987, when the first survey was administered to the sample of teachers, 57 out of 557, or approximately 10 percent, refused to complete the attitudinal survey. Reasons given for not completing the survey included such statements as: "I don't know enough about AIDS"; "I don't know anyone who has been infected with the AIDS virus"; and "My school doesn't have to worry about AIDS." On the other hand, when the second survey was administered only 7 out of 400, or approximately 2 percent, refused to complete the survey. Also, the administrators of the survey indicated that the respondents were much more physically relaxed while answering the questions and seem more confident in their responses. This confidence in their responses was evidenced by less embarrassment and fewer indications of nervousness. The overall comfort level of the 1991 teachers is further evidenced by the fact that in 1987, the overall time to complete the survey was 22 minutes whereas in 1991 the average time was less than 10 minutes.

In summary, results of the survey indicate that the overall attitude of the 1991 teachers was less negative towards AIDS than that of the 1987 teachers. Also, where differences were found between males and females, the males were consistently more negative towards the issues than the females. This finding might be explained by the fact that AIDS has been predominantly considered to be a male disease.

In the analysis relative to age, it was found that the 36–45 age group of teachers felt more strongly that they should not be required to teach students with AIDS than those teachers whose age was less than 36. The data in this survey provide no suggestion as to why these age group differences occurred.

Relative to the concept of issuing a teaching certificate to a person who tested positive for AIDS but showed no outward signs, those teachers who identified themselves as kindergarten through ninth grade teachers were more likely to agree with issuing the certificate than the teachers in the K–12 area. However, when asked if infected students should *not* be allowed to participate in school activities, these same K–12 teachers were the ones who most strongly disagreed with the item. The 7–9 teachers were more likely to agree than the K–12 teachers that teachers should not be required to teach students with AIDS. Although there are significant differences in the responses to a few of the items, the results do not provide a clear pattern of responses relative to the grade level at which the teachers were teaching.

Also, the survey indicates that there is very little difference in the responses to the items among those teachers who hold a bachelor's degree, fifth year certification, or a master's degree. However, those teachers with a master's degree did feel more strongly that teachers should not be required to teach students infected with AIDS.

Finally, continued research needs to be conducted with larger samples and populations on a regular basis in order to provide professionals with evidence that their collaborative efforts are indeed affecting the attitudes of teachers. The spread of AIDS will continue to be a critical issue that will challenge most educators. Since teachers must make personal decisions regarding their attitudes and beliefs, we must provide them with the most current and accurate information available regarding AIDS so they can address the issue meaningfully. Teachers have a powerful influence on their students, and the attitudes they convey to those students will set the stage for future generations.

Part II
Facing the Challenge

Chapter Nine

Placement of Students with HIV in Public Schools: Policy Considerations for Educators

WEMME E. WALLS

In recent years with the passage of the Education of the Handicapped Act (1975) public schools have greatly expanded programs for children with special educational needs. However, educational programs and policies have not yet met the particular health and educational needs of children with chronic illness (Hobbs, 1985). Identification and protection of chronically ill children as a "group" with guarantees and protections of the EHA has been difficult and continues to be controversial. The issues that are specific policy questions for the chronically ill child encompass specific issues which are as controversial for the child with human immunodeficiency virus (HIV) infection. Due to the additional concerns of health and safety to others, the educational placement of HIV-infected children involves a myriad of issues facing regular education and special education administrators and educators, and public health officials.

This chapter will focus on developments in medicine and in the courts that may have crucial implications for existing policies related to the educational placement issues of the HIV-infected student. A review of the salient medical and legal aspects related to the educational placement issues of school attendance for children with HIV is presented to provide information that will serve as a resource to public school personnel who are among the professionals that must make informed decisions on public school attendance policies for students with a lethal, complex, and controversial disease. Recommendations for decision and policy making will be discussed including awareness of pertinent state education, civil rights, and public health law; establishment of a vehicle for maintaining a network of resources for disseminating and implementing new information; knowledge of existing public educational policies at national, state, and local levels to support educational policy and decision making that is reasonable and sound; and issues of confidentiality and the infected child's right to privacy. Policy considerations will be reviewed to serve as an information resource for school officials to enable them to make informed proactive decisions. The chapter reviews results of a research study that includes medical evidence that supports policies on admission or exclusion of HIV-infected students in the public schools; an analysis of the relevant legal issues of the Education of the Handicapped Act (EHA), Section 504 of the Rehabilitation Act of 1973, and constitutional issues pertinent to educational placement of HIV-infected children; and case law "in point" or "analogous" to the issues addressed.

HIV as a Public School Issue

Infection by HIV has emerged as a serious public health problem in the United States. It is an issue of social, political, medical, economic, and legal controversy. Mass media coverage and the growing complexity of scientific information present a confusing picture to the public at large. Media coverage of AIDS is discussed further in Chapter Three. Issues surrounding the educational placement of public school children who are identified with HIV are equally controversial, complex, and confusing to educators and school officials who are responsible to the communities that support local educational agencies (LEAs). School officials are placed in a position of balancing the duty to protect the health and safety of the students and the duty to protect the system.

Transfusion-associated and perinatal transmission cases of AIDS and HIV account for a small percentage of overall cases in the United States, though the numbers continue to rise dramatically. Approximately 1.6 percent of the CDC-reported cases of AIDS are among infants, children, and adolescents. (Although the percentage is small when looking at overall numbers of reported AIDS cases, the numbers are expected to continue to increase dramatically [Baltimore and Wolff, 1986; Phair, 1987].)

The appearance of HIV cases in children and the well-publicized issue of school attendance for several of these children is of concern to public health, school health and school officials faced with the educational placement decisions of an issue that has attracted community interest and concern. The fear of the unknown can have serious legal, ethical, and social ramifications. The public schools are in a unique position to assume a role in providing to staff, pupils, parents, and the community both an awareness and interest in one of the most complex issues of the decade.

Medical experts in the field of AIDS research generally support the assumption that HIV infection is not transmitted easily or casually. However, controversy continues as to the solidity of this assumption, causing a potential for continual misunderstandings in dealing with the disease and the individuals infected. Some school systems have understandably resisted accepting the assurances of the medical profession in developing policies on procedures for educational placement of children with the virus (Weiner, 1986). Such resistance, while understandable to a degree, has not been encouraged by the courts. In the tragic and much publicized case of the Ray brothers of Florida, the court held that denial of access to the school setting was unacceptable. The Ray family received a $1.1 million settlement award from the school district (*Ray v. School District,* 1987). Few school districts will risk the exclusion of students with HIV "knowing that such a liability is possible" (Murphy, 1990).

Local community constraints and political controls complicate the decision-making process. Issues differentiating the rural school setting from the urban setting may also add to the complexities. Geographic isolation, informal systems of communication and lack of availability of professional resources are among the many additional issues that the educator must address when considering policy for educational placement of the HIV-infected student. Although many school districts have developed policies based on immediate need, many communities have acted in a proactive manner, anticipating that inevitably a child or children with HIV will be attending their schools. The "inevitability" continues to become more apparent, in part due to the movement of the virus into the heterosexual community, which has increased the numbers of those infected with the virus thus increasing the numbers of children contracting HIV through perinatal transmission.

The HIV infection is not known or suspected to have been transmitted from one child to another in schools, day-care, or foster-care settings. Transmission would necessitate exposure to the blood or other body fluids of an infected child, a highly unlikely occurrence in the school environment. Routine safety procedures for handling blood or other body fluids are effective in preventing transmission from children with the HIV infection to other children in classroom settings (Koop, 1986). Therefore, schools need no special precautions to protect others in the environment from possible transmission of the virus with exception of the adoption of routine precautions for handling blood and body fluids in cases of accident or injury. The state of Connecticut was among the first to develop educational policy issues that specifically address health care precautions. Their procedural manual has been used widely as a prototype for the handling of blood and other bodily fluids. (It is important to note that in 1988 the CDC revised guidelines for health care workers clarifying that universal precautions did not apply to feces, nasal secretions, sputum, sweat, tears, urine, or vomitus unless there was also a visible presence of blood.)

The National CDC guidelines first issued in August of 1985 recommended that, in most cases, school-age children with HIV be allowed to enter or remain in school. The CDC suggested that restrictive environments *may* be appropriate for preschool children, children with open lesions, or children lacking control of body secretions who are HIV-infected. In addition to the health and safety guidelines, the CDC recommendations recognize that there are legal issues to be considered in forming guidelines for the education of HIV-infected children, including the constitutional rights of the individual, the protection of children with disabilities under the EHA and Section 504 of the Rehabilitation Act of 1973, and the confidentiality of student's school records under the Family Education Rights and Privacy Act (FERPA) of 1974 and the regulations for EHA. National education groups such as the National Education Association, American Federation of Teachers, and the Council of Exceptional Children have existing policies on HIV and educational placement issues of HIV-infected students that parallel National Centers for Disease Control (CDC) recommendations of case-by-case decision making (Weiner, 1986).

Legal Issues of Educational Placement

Legal actions over issues paralleling the CDC guidelines were brought in Indiana, New York, and New Jersey by parents and others concerned with the school attendance of children diagnosed with AIDS (*White v. Western School Corp.,* 1985; *District 27 v. Board of Education of the City of New York,* 1985; *Board of Education of the City of Plainfield v. Cooperman,* 1985). To date, the courts have generally held that children with HIV should be permitted to attend school unless attendance of the child is contrary to reasonable medical judgments of the child's physician and or public health officials. Analogous cases involving school attendance of children with herpes simplex virus (HSV) and hepatitis B virus (HBV) have been previously resolved in favor of infected children who were seeking entrance to classrooms (*Council Bluffs Education Association v. Council Bluffs Community School District,* 1984; *New York Association for Retarded Children v. Carey,* 1979; *Community High School District #155 v. Denz,* 1984).

In November of 1986, the first decision of a case "in point" concerning a school attendance case was decided by a federal court in California. The court held that AIDS was a protective handicap under Section 504 of the Rehabilitation Act of 1973, so the school district involved in the suit was required to "reasonably accommodate" the child's handicap. Additionally, the court held that the school district failed to show that the child presented a risk to others, rejecting 1985 CDC guidelines that suggest biting as high risk behavior which may require a more restrictive environment (*Thomas v. Atascadero,* 1986). The *Atascadero* ruling is of greatest significance to educational placement issues due to the court's interpretation of the "significant risk of transmission" standard under Section 504 (Murphy, 1990).

Issues in HIV litigation and legislation that have influenced school attendance decisions include the exclusion of children not identified with AIDS or HIV infection, but in household contact with the virus (Matthews and Neslund, 1987; Weiner, 1986), and cases of children who were asymptomatic carriers of HIV and encountered difficulties in attending school (*Phipps v. Saddleback,* 1986; *Ray v. School District,* 1987).

The virus has already had a profound effect on the United States medical community. The growing array of cases and legislation indicates that AIDS-related legal issues in the public health and education sectors have had significant influence in public school policy and decision making as it concerns placement of children with HIV in public school classrooms. The controversy that surrounds educational placement in the public schools of children with HIV continues, as medical and legal issues unfold.

School officials are often unaware of court decisions and the implications of those decisions on problem solving, decision making, and policy issues. Some school officials have been faced with the additional burden of making decisions and policy recommendations relating to an issue on which there has been no previous policy, and in the absence of conclusive information on the medical and legal aspects of the concern. Medical evidence is a crucial factor in determining risk transmission. As the Supreme Court held in *School Board of Nassau County v. Arline* (1987), reasonable medical judgments must be considered.

A widely publicized example of a potential dilemma facing school systems related to the emerging issue of HIV and its broader counterpart, "communicable disease," was the Kokomo, Indiana, case of *White v. Western School Corp.* (1985). In defending the policy of excluding the 14-year-old from the classroom, school officials supported a position that was consistent with communicable disease law in the state, "although the state had issued guidelines directing schools to admit most students with the AIDS virus" (Weiner, 1986). In most public health state policy, HIV is not considered under communicable disease law and procedures due to the transmission factors. Ryan White's case became a focal point for many later policy decisions on educational placement of students with HIV.

There is a need to clarify existing laws and to anticipate emerging laws that impact upon the determination of educational placement of children with HIV. Litigation on AIDS is a previously uncharted area of law. The study of emerging precedents and patterns provides information that enables school officials to discern the basis for the decisions rendered or the possible course of action that might be anticipated in future disputes. In delineating precedents and patterns, school officials are able to make reasonable, informed, proactive decisions that will promote preventative law and policy that will be both cost-effective and time-efficient to the educational system.

Decision makers should be familiar with medical evidence and legal issues that may both directly and indirectly affect policy. Informed school personnel provide the impetus for the establishment and continuance of positive, well-developed dialogue among staff, students, parents, and the community.

While there is no medical evidence to support the exclusion of children from regular school attendance based on suspicion or identification of the HIV infection, in presenting medical evidence for the establishment of policy in educational decision making, it must be stressed that the nature of the information is dynamic. Individuals involved in and responsible for policy decision must keep abreast of new developments as they are reported, in order to provide accurate information and knowledgeable leadership. Recommendations on school attendance issued by the Centers for Disease Control (CDC) and the American Academy of Pediatrics (AAP) provide guidelines that suggest that some students with HIV may pose a greater risk than others and a more restrictive environment may be warranted for those students. These guidelines and recommendations provide a basis for arguing that there is minimal risk of transmission of the HIV infection in casual settings, such as the classroom.

In 1987, the *Report of the Surgeon General's Workshop on Children with HIV Infection and Their Families* issued recommendations that support the existing CDC and AAP guidelines as adequate resources in most respects with modifications suggested as they relate to the preschool population. In the report it is noted that "it should become possible for AIDS to be considered with neither more or less emotion than other severe illness of infancy and childhood. Key issues of epidemiology are poorly understood by most segments of society. A concerted community effort should be undertaken..." (Recommendation 8). Well-informed school officials responsible for policies and procedures on educational placement are in the best position to educate and inform parents, children, and staff of an issue that is often misunderstood. Awareness of sound medical evidence to support educational decision making provides a means of projecting well-grounded information to the school population and community at large.

Further study is needed in the area of medical aspects of placing students with HIV in the classroom. Efforts need to be made to isolate the unique needs of the high risk groups specific to childhood and adolescence, such as sexually abused individuals and substance abusers. Adolescents represent a unique subset of individuals whose specific needs must be addressed in communicating the circumstances surrounding transmission and contraction of the virus. Additional topics needing study include the implications of the disproportionate number of urban and minority children and adolescents infected with or at risk for transmission of the HIV infection and the impact the spread of the virus will have on these groups, medically and educationally. Mass media coverage of noted individuals, such as athletes Magic Johnson and Arthur Ashe, may provide the much needed exposure HIV warrants. While media coverage in itself was controversial regarding the announcements of both Ashe and Johnson, the upsurgence of interest in HIV has again brought the issue to the forefront. (More discussion on media coverages of AIDS is provided in Chapter Three.)

Renewed concern toward issues of confidentiality has also emerged. Protection of an individual's right to privacy is often overlooked in favor of public interest. A comparison of attitudes and perceptions between school personnel in districts that have direct need to know policies for all individuals responsible for the education of the HIV-infected student and those who have strict confidentiality with complete anonymity is suggested as one measure to evaluate the degree of stigma and fear that may be associated with the issue.

Emerging legal issues presented by the AIDS controversy primarily focus on the aspects of educational placement and provision of services for children in the public schools with the HIV infection. Of significance are the constitutional issues of equal protection and right to association, the determination of qualifying handicap under Section 504, and the application of the EHA to children with AIDS or the HIV infection. School personnel should be advised that while an HIV-infected student is not deemed disabled under EHA, the HIV-infected student is deemed as "handicapped" for purposes of protection under Section 504.

Section 504

Federal judicial interpretations support the content that AIDS and the HIV infection qualify as a protected handicap under Section 504 of the Rehabilitation Act, indicating that an automatic exclusion policy of children with the HIV infection from public schools should be viewed as a violation of Section 504 and its implementing regulations. The Supreme Court ruling in 1987 of *School Board of Nassau County v. Arline* (107 S. Ct. 1123) held that AIDS did qualify as a "physical impairment" for purposes of the Rehabilitation Act. Risk of contagion had been a major obstacle in the attainment of protected status until the 1987 *Arline* ruling. In declaring AIDS as a handicap, Schumaker (1986) suggests that persons received as having HIV, in addition to those with the actual disease, could find legal refuge in the anti-discrimination law.

The EHA defines "handicap" more narrowly than Section 504 and not all children deemed "handicapped" for purposes of Section 504 will necessarily qualify as "other health impaired" (OHI) under EHA. Human immunodeficiency virus may or may not be considered as a "communicable disease" under state law and may or may not be considered "OHI," dependent upon state definitional criteria.

For most purposes of the programming under the EHA, children with HIV are not educationally disabled merely because of the illness. The status of the child in regard to special programs depends upon the ability to perform in the regular classroom without adverse effects. If it is determined that a child with

HIV requires special education services, EHA regulations apply. Although the EHA recognizes that not all children may be placed in a normal school environment, the statute does require that a decision not to mainstream be justified by evidence that reflects the child's special needs. When a placement decision is made solely on the basis of the student's HIV status, the precedent has been set for bypassing EHA administrative remedies and proceeding under 504 as a discriminatory action. In *Martinez v. School Board* (1988), after lengthy court battles over exclusion of a child with neurological injury from a TMH self-contained classroom, the district court held that while both parties were of agreeance to her programming, there was an obvious dispute over safety issues and risk of transmission. Therefore, the issue became not appropriateness of program, but whether the child was being discriminated against due to her handicapping condition.

State Policy and Constitutional Issues

State administrative guidelines, with the exception of the regulatory status of procedures in Pennsylvania and New Jersey, are primarily advisory in nature. Local education agencies have the primary responsibility for establishing educational policies and procedures on the issue. Individuals responsible for policy decisions should be familiar with state and national trends that may directly or indirectly affect policy.

Medical evidence at the present time strongly suggests that policies of exclusion will not hold up constitutionally under the equal protection clause of the Fourteenth Amendment since no rational basis for excluding children from public school settings exists unless individual circumstances warrant the exclusion. Additionally, implementation of an exclusionary policy would probably be considered more intrusive than necessary and may be considered an infringement of property and freedom of association rights. As medical knowledge continues to emerge, justification for infringement upon the fundamental rights of the individual may shift. In the school environment the balance must be made between the rights of the individual to participate in school programs weighed against the potential of harm to others in the same environment.

Recommendations for Policy

The spread of AIDS is a topic of medical, legal, social, economic, and educational speculation and concern. The educational decision maker must be knowledgeable in communicating well-informed policy in educational issues concerning this topic. The service provider must have a strong vehicle of communication to translate information in the community setting. A network of resources should be developed and a vehicle put in place for disseminating and implementing new information as it develops.

The following are general recommendations for the educational decision maker in determining educational placement policy of students with HIV in the public schools.

- In developing and administering policy, school administrators should establish and maintain open communication with the major policy and rule-makers in the state. Knowledge of existing public agency policies at the national, state, and local levels supports educational policy that is sound and reasonable. Direction of HIV policy may be under the jurisdiction of education officials, public health officials, or both. Interagency collaboration is crucial to efficient, concise, and accurately administered policy recommendations.
- The National Centers for Disease Control (CDC) recommendations on the educational placement of students with HIV provide a guide when developing eligibility criteria for admission or exclusion of students in the public schools. In the school environment the rights of the individual to participate in school programs must be weighed against the potential of harm to others in the school environment. Medical evidence does not support exclusion of the student with HIV from public school classrooms. Potential harm to others in the public schools is not considered significant and in the majority of circumstances does not outweigh the rights of the individual to regular classroom placement.
- Although state laws may differ as to the interpretation on whether the child with HIV should be covered by EHA, it is suggested that school policy determine information on the responsible agent for education of children with HIV within the schools, be it regular or special education.
- Statutory and regulatory requirement of the EHA and Section 504 of the Rehabilitation Act provide guidance for policy and decision making concerning educational placement issues. The use of EHA procedures for case-by-case determination to provide clarity in decision making is suggested. However, in utilization of EHA procedures it is advisable to specify whether the use is for convenience or as a basis of eligibility for special education services.
- Routine precautions should be followed by all school personnel regardless of the presence or absence of an individual with HIV. There is no guarantee that knowledge of the individual with HIV will increase precaution. An open usage policy under which all school personnel are trained in precautionary procedures provides a vehicle for a safe school environment allowing for strict confidentiality to be maintained in an attempt to respect the child's right to privacy, if an HIV-infected student is present in the local public schools or district.

- Case-by-case review, as recommended in CDC guidelines, is suggested to determine if there is anything in the child's neurological, physical, or emotional behavior that would make an unrestricted environment inappropriate. Suggested panel review might entail two aspects: (a) determination that the child is well enough to attend school without undue risk to self, and (b) determination that the child's behavior does not pose an increased risk of transmission of HIV to others in the classroom. Composition of the panel should include representatives of medical, public health, and educational agencies within the community. There is no evidence that identification of the infected child is necessary for determination of placement status. A procedure should be in place for periodic review.
- Special education referral is suggested, only after panel review, if there is a determination that the physical condition of the child may have or has had an adverse effect on the child's learning.
- The number of persons knowledgeable of an infected child's condition should be kept at a minimum with disclosure only to those with a direct need to know. School policies and procedures that argue for disclosure of identity as a precautionary safeguard are not necessarily consistent with medical evidence that suggests routine safety procedures are effective in preventing the transmission of HIV. The decision of whether or not to disclose information regarding the student with HIV is most appropriately placed with those responsible for the protection of the child's health (e.g., the parents and the child's physician).
- Awareness of sound medical evidence to support educational decision making provides a means of projecting solidly grounded policy to the school and community at large. Depending on district size, a means of information-gathering should be in place to provide continuous updating of both medical and legal issues related to the educational placement of students with HIV. A network of resources should be developed for disseminating and implementing new information as it develops.

References

Baltimore, D., and Wilff, S. M., chairs (1986). *Confronting AIDS: Directions for Public Health, Health Care, and Research* (Institute of Medicine/National Academy of Sciences Report). Washington, DC: National Academy Press.

Blanchet, K. D. (1988). *AIDS: A Health Care Management Response.* Rockville, MD: Aspen Publications.

Hobbs, N., and Perrin, J. M., eds. (1986). *Issues in the Care of Children with Chronic Illness.* San Francisco: Jossey-Bass Publishers.

Koop, E. (1986). "Surgeon General's Report on Acquired Immune Deficiency Syndrome." *Journal of the American Medical Association,* 256(20):2783–2789.

Matthews, G. W., and Neslund, V. S. (1987). "The Initial Impact of AIDS on Public

Health Law in the United States." *Journal of the American Medical Association,* 257(3):344–352.

Murphy, M. M. (1990). "Special Education Children with HIV Infection: Standards and Strategies for Admission to the Classroom." *Journal of Law and Education,* 19: 345–370.

Phair, J. P., and Rapoza, N. P. (1987). "The Challenge of AIDS for Physicians Today: Information on AIDS for the Practicing Physician." *Monographs of the American Medical News,* 30 (2) (Suppl. 1).

Schumaker, A. M. (1986). "AIDS: Does It Qualify as a 'Handicap' Under the Rehabilitation Act of 1973?" *Notre Dame Review,* 61(3):572–594.

Weiner, R. (1986). *AIDS: Impact on the Schools.* Arlington, VA: Capital Publications, Inc.

Table of Cases

Board of Education of Plainfield v. Cooperman (A-1378-85T5) (N.J. Sup. Crt., App. Div., 1986).

Community High School District #155 v. Denz, 463 N.E.2d 998 (Ill. App. 1984).

Council Bluffs Education Ass'n v. Council Bluffs Community School Dist. (S.D. Iowa, 1984).

District 27 Community School Board v. Board of Education (Sup. Ct. N.Y. Queens County, 1986).

Martinez v. School Board, 861 F.2d 1502 (11th Cir. 1988).

Phipps v. Saddleback Unified School District, No. 474981 (Orange City Sup. Ct., 1986).

Ray v. School Dist., 666 7. Supp. 1524 (M.D. Fla. 1987).

School Board of Nassau v. Arline, 107 S. Ct. 1123 (1987), affirmed Arline v. School Board of Nassau, 172 F.2d 759 (11th Cir. 1985).

Thomas v. Atascadero Unified School District No. 886-609AHS (C.D. Calif., 1986).

White v. Western School Corporation (S.D. Ind., 1985).

Chapter Ten

Guidelines for HIV and AIDS Student Support Services

WORKING GROUP

The last decade has seen a convergence of factors that have changed public schools in profound ways. The rise of single parent families, the increasing diversity of the school population with growing numbers of immigrant students and students with limited English proficiency, the drug epidemic, and the high school dropout rate have now combined with the devastating impact of AIDS. Schools are challenged as never before to provide new and more comprehensive services to their students.

The purpose of the guidelines set forth in this chapter is to encourage schools to enhance the academic and social growth of all students through the effective delivery of HIV-related student support services. Although these services are not necessarily new, they do require additional efforts to assess student needs and to marshal resources. Services related to HIV will be most effective when they are incorporated into the framework of a comprehensive support services program which serves all students.

These guidelines set standards for the effective delivery of these services. Student support services personnel—such as school counselors, school nurses,

This chapter was developed by a Working Group of representatives from the American Association for Counseling and Development; American School Health Association; American Federation of Teachers; American Psychological Association; National Association of School Nurses; National Association of School Psychologists; National Association of Social Workers, Education Commission; National Association of State School Nurse Consultants; and National Coalition of Advocates for Students. Additional endorsing organizations are Midwest School Social Work Services; and National Education Association Health Information Network. Funding was provided by a cooperative agreement (#U63/CCU102809-04) with the Division of Adolescent and School Health, Center for Chronic Disease Prevention and Health Promotion, Centers for Disease Control.

school psychologists, and school social workers—can work with health educators, teachers, administrators, aides, and other school staff to help students understand the impact of the HIV epidemic on their lives, guide them to adopt or maintain healthy behaviors, and provide support to those dealing personally with HIV infection.

Many schools will not have a full complement of personnel to student support services. Budgetary constraints in many districts have meant heavy caseloads and assignment of individual support service personnel to multiple school sites. When this is the case, teachers, administrators, and paraprofessional staff can, with sufficient training and administrative support, provide many of the support services outlined in this document.

These guidelines describe a desirable multidisciplinary mix of student support services related to the HIV epidemic. They can be used by student support services personnel to evaluate the quality of service they are providing, by school administrators to design a comprehensive student support service delivery program, and by parents and child advocates to hold schools accountable for providing high quality support services. A checklist for evaluating HIV student support services appears at the end of the chapter.

Confidentiality

These support services involve the participation of many school staff. The identity of HIV-infected students and of those with HIV-infected family members must, however, be kept strictly confidential.

These guidelines do not broaden in any way the definition of who within a school has a need to know. In many instances, no student support service staff member has a need to know the identity of an HIV-infected student. A decision to increase the number of school staff who know the HIV status of a student or of a member of a student's family in order to receive support services must rest entirely with the infected student and his or her family. If a family decides to share this information with a school staff member, it is the duty of the staff person to keep the student's identity strictly confidential. Any written information about a student's HIV status should be kept in a secure location separate from the student's academic and other school records.

There may be occasions when a student will reveal his or her HIV status, or that of a family member, to a staff person. It should be emphasized that, in such a situation, the school staff member has a responsibility to explain to the student the possible risks and benefits of further disclosure. All school districts should immediately adopt and put into place a clear policy on the school attendance of HIV-infected students that includes strict limitations on who within the school system has a need to know the identity of such a student.

HIV and Youth

Adolescents are a primary risk group for HIV infection:

- Between January 31, 1989, and February 1, 1990, the number of cases among 13- to 19-year-olds increased by 40 percent (CDC, 1990b; CDC, 1989a: 12).
- Twenty percent of people reported with AIDS have been between the ages of 20 and 29 (CDC, 1990b: 12). With an incubation period of up to 10 years or more, many were infected in their teenage years.
- An even ratio of males to females diagnosed with AIDS is generally considered an indication of heterosexual transmission (CDC, 1989b). The overall ratio among U.S. adults is ten males to one female. Among teenaged military recruits, this ratio is reduced to 1.09 males to 1 female (Burke et al., 1990).
- Fifty-three percent of all teenagers reported with AIDS have been African-American or Latino (CDC, 1990b: 12), although African-American and Latino teenagers make up only about 21 percent of the U.S. adolescent population (National Research Council, 1987).

Teenagers exhibit behaviors that result in a high incidence of sexually transmitted diseases (STDs). These same behaviors place a person at risk for HIV infection.

- By age 19, 63 percent of females and 78 percent of males have had sexual intercourse (Center for Human Resource Research, 1983).
- Of sexually active U.S. females, those aged 10–19 years have the highest rate of gonorrhea (Hein, 1989).
- At least one in every five American males has had sex with another male in which he or his partner came to orgasm. Of these men, 93.3 percent had such an experience when they were aged 19 or younger (Fay et al., 1989).

The use of illegal drugs increases the risk of HIV infection among some teenagers. In four urban sites, 3.7–6.7 percent of students aged 13–18 years reported having injected cocaine, heroin, or other illegal drugs at some time in their lives (CDC, 1988). All drug use—alcohol, crack, and intravenous—impairs judgment and may contribute heavily to high risk sexual behavior. Additionally, some teenagers engage in prostitution to support their drug addictions.

The Need for HIV-Related Student Support Services

Student support services include social, psychological, health, and other services delivered to students by school nurses, school psychologists, school counselors, and social workers. There will be times, however, when school administrators, teachers, aides, and other school personnel will also deliver support services to students. Recognizing that classroom learning and academic achievement are strongly influenced by a student's physical and emotional health, economic status, and home and community environments, these services typically include health screening, short-term psychological and vocational counseling, referral to community agencies for social services needed by students and their families, and psychological assessment.

Although the work is often educational in nature, support services are usually delivered outside the formal classroom. Maximum service delivery requires close collaboration among student support service personnel, health educators, other classroom teachers, administrators, and parents. School personnel have a responsibility to serve all students, regardless of race, sex, religion, sexual orientation, language, behavior, or learning style.

The AIDS epidemic underscores the importance of some ongoing student support services and creates a need for additional ones. Many of these services are educational and can be partially met by instructional programs. Student support services personnel can reinforce and supplement classroom teaching.

All students now need the following services:

- Factual information on the prevention of HIV infection.
- Access to school and community-based physical and mental health services.
- Counseling concerning adolescent development, sexuality, identity formation, peer pressure, and death and dying.
- Skills in communication, assertiveness, decision making, and problem solving.
- Peer acceptance of a range of healthy sexual attitudes and behaviors; this can be fostered and encouraged by school staff.
- Help in recognizing personal vulnerability to HIV infection.
- A supportive environment in which to express fears and anxiety about HIV infection.

Barriers to Effective Support Service Delivery

A number of obstacles may impede optimal delivery of HIV-related student support services. These can include the following:

- Lack of agreement among school staff, local boards of education and others that it is the school's role to provide a wide range of support services to students.
- Insufficient funding of student support service programs, resulting in heavy caseloads and assignment of individual service personnel to multiple school sites.
- Lack of implementation of support service delivery standards, inconsistent educational requirements for support service personnel, and ineffective monitoring of service quality.
- Inadequate pre-service and in-service training in the developing of skills supporting effective collaboration with other school personnel.
- Inadequate collaboration and coordination with community-based organizations.
- Inadequate administrative and institutional support.
- Inadequate implementation and evaluation of innovative student support service delivery models.
- Lack of coordination between various federal, state, and local programs, resulting in, for example, complex reporting requirements.
- Inadequate in-service training on new approaches to support service delivery and comprehensive school health education.
- Inadequate pre-service and in-service training which helps increase staff comfort discussing issues about sexuality and HIV infection.

Essential Components of an HIV Student Support Services Program

Prevention Education Education for HIV prevention must take place both in and out of the classroom. Student support services personnel should be involved at all levels: planning, development, implementation, and evaluation.

Prevention curricula must be skill-based and focused on experiential learning and on establishing positive health behaviors. Rather than emphasizing the medical aspects of HIV, curricula should teach skills in decision making, assertiveness, and communication. A curriculum that affirms sexuality as a positive, healthy aspect of human development is more likely to encourage young people to adopt positive health behaviors than a curriculum that uses language that judges and induces only fear. As recommended by the Centers for Disease Control and the Presidential Commission on the HIV Epidemic, HIV education should be carried out within a comprehensive health education program.

Education about preventing HIV infection should be infused into all HIV student support service programs. Student support service personnel are in a unique position to work with students individually and in small groups to translate classroom learning about HIV prevention into personal behavior change. By encouraging the development of decision making and communication skills and by counseling students on risk reduction, student support service personnel can help empower students to lead healthy lives. Student support services personnel can also play key roles in interpreting an HIV education program to parents and other members of the community. They can work with administrators and other school staff to promote comprehensive health education programs that include strong drug prevention and sexuality education components.

It is crucial that student support services personnel work closely with classroom teachers so that HIV prevention messages that are taught in the classroom can be reinforced in counseling and other settings; so that classroom teachers know where to turn to help students who express fears of HIV infection or who disclose sexual abuse; and so that student support services personnel are aware when classroom instruction concerning HIV, human sexuality and other sensitive health issues is occurring. These topics may lead some students to seek counseling and other support services.

Health-Related Services The school nurse should play a major role in assessing the health needs of an HIV-infected student and providing a safe and minimally restrictive environment within school. Confidentiality laws and guidelines should be observed in determining which school staff have a need to know of the student's HIV status.

Every HIV-infected student who has a special health care need requiring nursing care, intervention, monitoring or supervision during school hours should have a care plan written by a nurse. Such a nursing care plan is developed by the school nurse in collaboration with the student's primary health care provider with permission from the parent or guardian. The plan should clearly identify the specific health services needed, the school staff who will be responsible for providing the service, and the individual(s) who will train or supervise such staff. The plan should be evaluated and revised, as appropriate.

The health needs of an HIV-infected student differ from the needs of an HIV-infected adult. Pediatric AIDS often manifests itself as the development of severe bacterial infections, and a large proportion of infected children have mental or motor retardation. Comprehensive health care, however, has improved the quality of life and has resulted in fewer hospitalizations of infected youth. The need for health services during the school day will be increased, for instance, by the promising early results that indicate that drug treatment with AZT slows the replication of the virus. The development of other drugs that reduce bacterial infection will also increase the need for in-school health services. Health services, such as those listed below, should be provided by a school nurse, the school physician or professional staff in a school-based clinic and may include administration of medication, including AZT, aerosolized pentamidine and TB chemoprophylaxis; nutritional assessment and special feeding programs, including fine and gross motor coordination and maintenance of bowel and bladder control; and health counseling related to academic, peer, and family concerns.

The school psychologist should closely monitor the cognitive functioning of an HIV-infected student. Cognitive symptoms such as impaired memory, difficulty in visual-motor integration, poor concentration and problem solving, slowing of motor activity, emotional ability, and impaired intellectual functioning are associated with the progression of AIDS in pediatric cases. These symptoms could be noted through behavioral observation and standardized assessment procedures. A change in cognitive or emotional status may require referral to the primary care provider for full evaluation. It may also necessitate the provision of new school-based services as well as revisions of the student's individualized educational plan.

With the permission of the HIV-infected student and his or her family, a specific student support staff person should be assigned responsibility for coordination of support services. Whenever a student's physical or mental health status changes, this staff person should notify the student's parent or guardian and primary care provider. Parents and primary care providers must be informed of changes in cognitive functioning and of health risks that may arise at school. The designated coordinator of support services for an individual student may be asked to monitor attendance to ensure that the educational needs of the student are met during periods of absenteeism.

Counseling and Support Student support services personnel must provide students with counseling and support (individually or in groups) concerning HIV-related issues. A counselor may address issues ranging from immediate health concerns to grief to undue anxiety over HIV infection. All counseling should reinforce prevention messages and help students adopt risk reduction behaviors.

The difficult issues facing adolescents, especially those related to sexual development, have been complicated by the existence of a usually fatal sexually transmitted disease. Counseling should be geared to an adolescent's cognitive abilities and be respectful of his or her cultural and religious background.

Counseling should be available for each of the following groups of students:

- AIDS symptomatic and HIV-positive students who were infected in utero or at birth, of whom an increasing number are remaining asymptomatic up to 8 to 9 years of age, as well as those infected by blood transfusions or blood products, unprotected sexual activity (either homosexual and heterosexual), sexual abuse, or sharing contaminated needles and syringes during intravenous drug use. These students need an effective advocate to prevent inappropriate placement in special education classes and to ensure adequate support services. Counseling is needed to address fears of stigmatization, decisions about revealing HIV-positive status, relationships to peers in social situations—especially dating—and issues of death and dying. Students who are symptomatic need assistance in managing medical treatment and coping with their changing health status.

- Students with family members or friends with AIDS need help coping with loss, guilt, denial, anger, and confusion. A student who may not know a family member has AIDS might pick up on the secrecy surrounding that person at home. School social workers and other student support services personnel can help parents assess student and family needs and identify community resources.
- Students who are gay or lesbian need a safe and confidential environment in which to discuss their fears and learn explicit risk-reduction behaviors. The HIV epidemic has intensified homophobia and has further isolated this group of already vulnerable youth.
- Students who are substance abusers need help in adopting drug and sexual behaviors that eliminate or reduce the risk of infection, as well as help in securing treatment for addiction.
- Students with limited English proficiency will need help from trained bilingual and bicultural staff to ensure that they receive the quality support services to which they are entitled. School staff should confirm that limited English proficient students understand the complexities and implications of the decisions they make about HIV issues.
- Students with physical or mental handicaps may have difficulty comprehending and attending to the message of HIV educational programs. Special efforts must be taken to ensure that appropriate support services are provided.
- Students with a history of sexually transmitted disease are at high risk for HIV infection. Not only can infection with an STD indicate unprotected sexual activity, some STDs may function as cofactors for HIV infection by facilitating transmission of the human immunodeficiency virus. School staff who treat students for STDs should provide counseling to such students on how to reduce the risk of contracting HIV and other STDs. Evidence of an STD should also trigger a referral to a counselor who is qualified to provide comprehensive HIV pretest and posttest counseling to adolescents.

Hiv Test Counseling and Support Students who consider HIV antibody testing face complex psychological and legal issues. Few test sites have counselors with experience in the special issues of adolescents at risk for HIV infection. It is important to note that pretest and posttest counseling available to adults may not be adequate for adolescents.

Counseling and support services must be available to any student who considers testing. This counseling must be comprehensive, culturally specific in the student's own language and geared to the student's cognitive abilities. Students must understand the difference between HIV infection and having AIDS, between anonymous and confidential test sites, and between false-negative and false-positive test results, as well as the importance of adopting risk reduction behaviors regardless of the test results. It is recommended that adolescents be tested in a site where ongoing follow-up medical and mental health care is available, such as an adolescent clinic, community health center, or a family planning clinic. The confidentiality of an adolescent considering or moving ahead with testing should be strictly guaranteed. Although not always statutorily explicit, legal authority exists in almost all states for physicians to test mature and competent adolescents without parental consent (North, 1990).

Students should be referred to a source of skilled counseling on adolescent testing issues rather than directly for testing. Comprehensive posttest counseling and medical follow-up must also be provided, including the identification of responsible adult support.

Where no sources exist for pretest and posttest counseling for adolescents, school personnel should work with community agencies to help develop such a capacity.

Some students who are especially worried about HIV infection may not have engaged in high risk behavior. Counseling may reveal other personal issues that are being manifested as undue anxiety over HIV infection.

Referral and Coordination of Support Services The provision of high quality student support services entails close cooperation between school staff and community youth-serving agencies. Student support service personnel are in a unique position to forge such a linkage since many share a common professional training and perspective with their counterparts in the community. Through referral networks and professional meetings, they should maintain ongoing contact with health providers, counselors, social workers and psychologists in community agencies. They must, however, be given the authority, time, resources, and administrative support to properly coordinate HIV-related student support services.

Student support services personnel should:

- *Identify resources.* Each school or district should designate a specific person to gather and update information on HIV services that are available to children, teenagers, and families in the community. School staff should identify organizations that provide home nursing, "buddies" for persons with AIDS, psychotherapy, emergency day care, HIV test counseling, support groups, drug treatment, and other assistance that might be needed by students and families dealing with HIV infection. When appropriate, referrals should be made to these services.
- *Create additional support service capacity.* When community resources

are inadequate, the school, as the primary youth-serving institution, should assume a leadership role in generating new support services at either the school or community level.

- *Coordinate support services to known HIV-infected and HIV-affected students.* Coordination of support services should begin with in-school resources, but should involve ongoing collaboration with a student's physician, with the health department, and with other social agencies that provide services to an HIV-nfected student. A designated student support service staff member should act as the primary coordinator of support services for an HIV-infected student who is symptomatic. If a student had difficulty coping with the HIV infection of a family member or friend, a designated school-based student support service staff member can be assigned to work with the student or the family to see that the family is referred to appropriate medical and social services in the community, that the student receives in-school counseling, and that understanding and support are available on a confidential basis.
- *Collaborate with community service agencies.* School and community agency staff must work together to establish effective linkages between school and community services. Moreover, the school must share joint responsibility with community agencies to ensure that the needs of students and families are met. To minimize community and school competition for scarce resources, school staff must place a high priority on building trust with community-based organizations. When both community agency and school staff stay focused on serving youth, competition and mistrust can be minimized.

Policymaking Student support service personnel should be involved at all levels in the formulation, implementation, and review of all policies concerning school attendance and the physical and mental health care of HIV-positive students during the school day. Many states have mandated HIV education or sex education either as part of a comprehensive health education program or as independent units. Many local school districts have already adopted specific school attendance policies. Development of these programs and policies, however, has not always included active participation by a full range of student support services personnel.

Student support services personnel can educate policymakers and the community about medically and psychosocially sound approaches to school attendance, HIV testing, confidentiality, in-school support services, and the effectiveness of universal infection control precautions. They can often contribute critical information about neighborhood and community conditions.

It is important to review existing policies to ensure that they reflect accurate information and research, that they designate individuals responsible for carrying out policies, and that they hold those individuals accountable for implementation.

Student support personnel should advocate at both state and local levels for strict guarantees of confidentiality and the formulation of policies based on accurate scientific information. Within the school system they should promote a team approach to the delivery of all support services. Teamwork entails an understanding of the services provided by various school-based personnel and a commitment on the part of all school staff members to work closely with each other to address student needs.

Staff Training Effective delivery of HIV-related student support services requires skilled, knowledgeable, and caring personnel. Student support services personnel must receive the proper training and administrative support to be able to demonstrate expertise in dealing with the issues posed by the HIV epidemic, including a thorough knowledge of how HIV is and is not transmitted, an understanding of adolescent growth and development, familiarity with the special issues HIV testing poses for teenagers, experience with successful strategies to help students make responsible decisions, and knowledge of relevant community services that may be needed by HIV-positive students and their families. They should also commit to a team model, developing a clear understanding of the services provided by their colleagues and working together to fully meet students' needs. Support personnel must be comfortable when discussing sensitive issues raised by the epidemic, such as teenage sexual behavior (including homosexual and bisexual behavior), drug use, and death and dying. And an important part of their jobs is to help schools adopt and enforce strict confidentiality guarantees. Children and adolescents are entitled to the same protection and standards as adults.

Two types of in-service training are essential. The first is simply a matter of informing support personnel of all available facts about HIV and AIDS. All school staff should understand how HIV is transmitted and how infection can be prevented. They should know where to get more information and help and understand universal infection control procedures.

The second kind of training needed is instruction for teaching and providing counseling and other services to students. Training staff for teaching or counseling is more rigorous than an informational in-service. In addition to learning accurate and detailed knowledge about HIV, participants need the chance to process the information in a way that alleviates their own fears of exposure to the virus. Staff members should be helped to examine their own attitudes about AIDS, sexuality, homosexuality, death, and other sensitive issues. Classroom and counseling strategies should be presented, including models for integrating HIV prevention into comprehensive health education programs. Training should enable staff to identify specific student behaviors they want to influence and to teach skills that students need to establish behaviors that reduce risk. The training itself should be skill-based—that is, staff members should be taught the skills they will then teach their students.

The school nurse and other medical staff should be trained to recognize the manifestations of HIV disease. They should also be trained to administer the medications or treatments HIV-infected students may need during the school day.

After comprehensive training, shorter in-service sessions should be held annually to update staff on new information about HIV infection and AIDS. All school districts should designate an individual to be responsible for monitoring new information about HIV infection. State-level student support organizations may be able to serve as a resource.

Checklist for Evaluating HIV Student Support Services

The following checklist can be used to evaluate the quality of school-based support services in relation to the HIV epidemic. In an effective service program, each question should elicit a "yes" answer.

- Is there an officially adopted policy that guarantees the right of HIV-infected students to attend school?
- Does the policy guarantee that the identity of the infected student will be kept confidential from all but the persons who have a professional need to know?
- Is each symptomatic HIV-infected student assigned to an appropriate student support staff member who secures needed services and coordinates school-based services with services in the community? (Note: If the designated coordinator is not someone who, under the school district's policy, would ordinarily have a need to know the identity of the infected student, permission from the student and his or her family must be obtained.)
- Are health care plans developed for students who need direct provision of health services in school?
- Is there a team approach to support service delivery among school staff?
- Are student support services personnel given sufficient resources to meet high standards of effective service provision?
- Are there enough personnel on staff to permit manageable caseloads for student support services personnel?
- Are student support services personnel given sufficient authority to monitor the provision of support services to HIV-infected students and to implement HIV-related policies?
- Arc gay and lesbian students offered counseling and prevention education that acknowledges their sexual orientation and that discusses same-gender sexual behavior and HIV risk reduction in straightforward, nonjudgmental ways?

- Are student support services personnel involved in all levels of planning, developing, implementing, and evaluating HIV prevention education programs?
- Are students with limited English proficiency provided quality HIV support services appropriate to their needs?
- Are handicapped students provided quality HIV support services appropriate to their needs?
- Are school staff aware of the range of health care, counseling, and other resources available in the community to HIV-infected children and teenagers and to their families?
- Is there administrative support for building strong linkages between school and community service providers?
- Is every student who considers HIV testing provided intensive counseling and follow-up support by a school or community-based counselor trained to work with adolescents on HIV testing issues?
- Are members of the school staff helped to examine their own attitudes about sexuality, HIV infection, and death and dying?
- Are school staff members given accurate and detailed information about HIV infection and AIDS?
- Are designated staff members trained to provide adequate health care services for HIV-infected students?
- Are designated staff trained to provide appropriate counseling for HIV-infected students and other students concerned about HIV issues?

References

Burke, D. S.; Brundage, J. F.; Goldenbaum, M.; Gardner, L. I.; Peterson, M.; Visintine, R.; Redfield, R. R.; and the Walter Reed Retrovirus Research Group (1990). "Human Immunodeficiency Virus Infections in Teenagers: Seroprevalence Among Applicants for U.S. Military Service." *JAMA,* 263:2075.

Center for Human Resource Research (1983). National Longitudinal Survey of Youth. Ohio State University.

Centers for Disease Control (1988). "HIV-Related Beliefs, Knowledge, and Behaviors Among High School Students." *Morbidity and Mortality Weekly Report,* 37:718.

____ (1989a, February). *HIV/AIDS Surveillance.*

____ (1989b). "Update: Heterosexual Transmission of AIDS and HIV Infection—U.S." *Morbidity and Mortality Weekly Report,* 38:423–433.

____ (1990a). "Estimates of HIV Prevalence and Projected AIDS Cases: Summary of a Workshop, October 31–November 1, 1989." *Morbidity and Mortality Weekly Report,* 39:117.

____ (1990b, March). *HIV/AIDS Surveillance.*

____ (1990c, February). *HIV/AIDS Surveillance.*

Fay, R. E.; Turner, C. F.; Klassen, A. D.; and Gagnon, J. H. (1989). "Prevalence and Patterns of Same-Gender Sexual Contact Among Men." *Science,* 243:338.

Hein, K. (1989). "AIDS in Adolescents: Exploring the Challenge." *Journal of Adolescent Health Care,* 10:20–21.

National Research Council (1987). *Risking the Future: Adolescent Sexuality, Pregnancy, and Childbearing.* Washington: National Academy Press, pp. 34–35.

North, R. L. (1990). "Legal Authority for HIV Testing of Adolescents." *Journal of Adolescent Health Care,* 11:185.

Chapter Eleven

Integrating Community-Based Resources into AIDS Education Curricula

A. ODASUO ALALI

School-based health clinics are having a significant impact on students' awareness and knowledge about sexuality and sexually transmitted diseases (STDs). In most cases, these school-based programs have been effective in disseminating information to America's youths about the human immunodeficiency virus (HIV) that causes acquired immunodeficiency syndrome (AIDS). Despite this improved student health knowledge, however, most programs offered by school-based clinics do not necessarily induce behavioral changes that would reduce students' chances to engage in risky behaviors that increase their chances of infection with HIV. Several factors contribute to this difficulty.

The major problem with achieving behavior change in students is not the result of information; the majority of young people understand how HIV is transmitted, yet deny or ignore their vulnerability. The problem, as Shayne and Kaplan (1988) observe, is that "educational programs about AIDS often fail to change attitudes or prejudices because they neglect consideration of the intense emotional reaction elicited by this syndrome" (p. 186). This observation is especially relevant because young people believe that public education programs about AIDS are misguided: "Nearly three-quarters of young people (72 percent) say that public education efforts to reduce the spread of AIDS among young people should focus more on encouraging them to practice safe sex than on encouraging them to abstain from sex (26 percent)" (Schmiedeskamp, 1991, p. 2).

Although educational approaches may not necessarily address the attitudinal problems of young people, "school is the optimal setting to launch AIDS education for young people. Schools have the potential to reach 95 percent of the nation's young people with this vitally important information" (Haffner, 1987, p. 5). The lack of appropriate teaching or educational materials in public schools, however, has affected AIDS education and prevention programs in schools. In short, the neglect of an essential teaching component will have a negative impact on the attainment of most public schools' education objectives.

In an analysis of what teachers in public schools teach about AIDS, STDs, and pregnancy prevention, Forrest and Silverman (1989) observed that even though "many teachers list student reactions or lack of interest as one of their most important problems, this may also be a reflection of the adequacy of available teaching materials and strategies" (p. 72). The unintended consequence, as articulated by Forrest and Silverman, is that "teachers must use valuable time to develop many teaching materials themselves. Because teachers are not experts in many of the topics they must cover, developing their own materials adds to the danger that dated, inaccurate information may be passed on to students" (p. 72).

Though 85 percent of the general public agree that public schools should offer sexuality education (Kanter, 1994, p. 7), an even greater number (nine in ten) parents (Haffner, 1994, p. 17) and 91 percent of the general public support teaching of AIDS prevention to children in public school (National Broadcasting Corporation, 1987). The reality, however, is that this yearning has not been equaled by deeds for teachers; they simply have not received the necessary support from government to achieve their education objectives in the age of AIDS. The fight against AIDS among teenagers in the United States is at the forefront of government neglect. A report by the House Select Committee on Children, Youth and Families acknowledged that "United States efforts to combat AIDS among young Americans are underfunded, uncoordinated and largely unsuccessful" ("AIDS in 13–24 Age Range," 1992, p. A-14). As supportive evidence, the report noted that "federal agencies that fight AIDS spent $107 million [in 1991], or 5 percent of the total AIDS-fighting budgets, on teenagers" (p. A-14).

An ancillary obstacle to AIDS education and prevention is fueled by the prejudice that is associated with the disease. From the onset, AIDS has been labeled by most people as a homosexual disease. This perception has developed into negative attitudes towards gay people. "Three in five (61 percent) of Americans surveyed feel the tolerance of gay life in the 1960s and 1970s was a 'bad thing for our society' " (Hugick & Leonard, 1991, p. 62). The residues of these attitudes are felt either in what governments can provide schools, in the shape AIDS curricula take, or in how students perceive their vulnerability to AIDS ("If it is a gay disease, then I cannot get it, because I'm heterosexual"). Lastly, it also seems that class differentials play a part in how AIDS information is disseminated, especially as seen in inner-city public schools whose student bodies are predominantly ethnic minorities (Alali, 1992). How can schools position themselves to address the emotional factors that interact with behavior change in young people? This chapter addresses that question by directing the attention of school health educators to community-based resources that would be invaluable to their AIDS education curricula. Clearly, this is important to health educators because single, school-based interventions simply have not worked and will not work. They should be linked with other community-based intervention programs. It is possible that students' attitudes toward AIDS will change, and their susceptibility to HIV will be clearly articulated to them, if collaborative efforts between public schools and community organizations reinforce young people's awareness of their vulnerability to the virus.

Community-Based Resources

There are numerous AIDS education resources that are located within the geographical areas of most public schools. These resources include services and activities that community-based organizations (CBOs) provide for effective health education to prevent the spread of HIV among youths. These organizations include churches, synagogues, community agencies, youth-service agencies, health care providers, and AIDS advocacy organizations. Their services range from speakers' bureaus to individual counseling and volunteer training (Bailey, 1991, p. 703). Community-based organizations primarily work informally with schools and other youth service agencies to prevent the spread of HIV among youths. The names, addresses, and relevant information about these CBOs can be obtained through state AIDS network groups, county health departments, or listings in the telephone book. One can also contact the National AIDS Information Clearinghouse at 1-800-458-5231 for referrals and reference assistance. The following sections examine the specific services of CBOs that can benefit public schools. For simplicity's sake, these services can be classified within five specific areas: information, education, training, support programs, and advocacy functions.

Information Through cooperative agreements with government agencies and philanthropic organizations, CBOs have developed an array of information networks that provide services such as newsletters, journals, brochures, fliers, and posters. In this capacity, most CBOs serve as clearinghouses for the exchange of information about AIDS and to coordinate AIDS information efforts. Because most of this information has been reviewed by experts in the field, they meet acceptable standards for education about AIDS.

Education Community-based organizations, most of which are voluntary nonprofit groups, have responded to the complex needs of those who need to know about HIV and those infected with the virus. Consequently, they have developed numerous educational services that can help schools achieve their educational objectives. There are four areas of educational services that public schools should consider integrating into their intervention programs.

First is technical assistance through curriculum and program development, implementation, and evaluation. Schools often design their curricula for use across a wide range of student ages without consideration of emotional factors, cultural issues, and the sociopolitical realities that affect their learning. Those CBOs that are not constrained by bureaucracies help schools develop AIDS curricula that are suitable for age and grade levels in variety of settings. These include activities that would accommodate immigrant students and lead to the development of a curriculum that is culturally relevant and sensitive to the student population, particularly in terms of Spanish and English versions.

Similarly, some CBOs are willing to fund the development of curricula, and to help schools design, implement, and evaluate the effectiveness of their HIV prevention programs. It is important that schools develop these collaborative relationships and partnerships with CBOs so that their curricula can be reviewed for scientific accuracy, and so they can assess the degree to which a given curriculum meets their educational needs. Such invaluable technical assistance may help schools provide their students with effective health education, particularly about AIDS.

The second area needing attention is the strengthening of available curriculum resource materials. One of the major problems educators face is the lack of AIDS curriculum resources to supplement their teaching materials; they are simply scarce or inaccessible to educators. Community-based organizations can bridge the gap that now exists by providing public schools with specific resource materials, such as interactive modules to teach students about decision making; helping schools identify sufficient resources to meet the needs of their HIV/AIDS education programs; and providing schools with updated, annotated computerized bibliographies of relevant educational materials, programs, research, and resources. Most CBOs that provide schools with resource materials are located within the geographical area of the schools they serve.

The third area is the development of workshops and seminars, which often provide discussions that serve as an opportunity to distribute educational materials and information that raises awareness of the AIDS issue. These workshops or seminars target not only teachers who must teach students about the disease, but also out-of-school and in-school youths. These workshops or seminars may be executed as part of an "AIDS awareness week" program. In the process, these activities increase general public awareness of AIDS as a critical children's issue. Also, they may reduce the threat of repercussions or discrimination against persons with AIDS.

The final area is peer education. These programs work to train young people in the content and methods of AIDS education and counseling so that they can serve as more responsible models to their peers; to correct myths and misinformation; to develop innovative peer approaches to teen pregnancy and HIV/AIDS prevention; to use peer pressure effectively (Center for Population Options [CPO], 1989, p. 7; CPO, 1983); to train teens to "become advocates and resources for other teens" (CPO, 1989, p. 9); and, most important, to help teens channel their energies in creating educational campaigns for their age group. A good example is the CPO's Teens for AIDS Prevention (TAP) programs, which has created AIDS campaign posters, buttons, rap songs, and school assemblies in Washington, D.C., and other cities. Similar programs may exist in the reader's community; their involvement in AIDS education curricula is recommended because "the message they deliver is direct and powerful in helping teens understand and respond to the threat of HIV infection" (CPO, 1989, p. 9).

Training Schools can also benefit from CBOs because the latter offer training programs to improve HIV-related knowledge, awareness, and counseling skills of teachers through train-the-trainer programs. In this role, teachers are trained about HIV infection and AIDS and in education of youth, how to incorporate HIV risk-reduction messages into activities provided to students, how to reach and intervene with students at risk and to prevent the spread of HIV infection, and how to discuss HIV and AIDS issues in a culturally relevant and sensitive way. Through this training, teachers become able to develop their own training modules and to help their schools create educational campaigns for students (including posters, buttons, rap songs, etc.). Also, the community at large, including parents, may gain from the training offered by CBOs.

Support Programs Community-based organizations can provide schools with support programs for out-of-school and in-school youths, as well as for persons with HIV or AIDS. These support services may include buddy programs, street outreach programs, telephone hotlines, individual and family counseling, and services that address the social and health needs of persons with AIDS. Additionally, CBOs can provide support services for gay and lesbian students that acknowledge their sexual orientation and aid in HIV risk reduction. Through these services, students often are able to meet with a person with AIDS who can provide them with a personal perspective about the disease.

Advocacy Community-based organizations serve an advocacy function for the school-age child. Consequently, governments depend on them for policy, because they research and document children's needs; they also develop progressive child welfare policies that emphasize protective guidelines. In the process, CBOs can link groups and other agencies on legal issues and educational reforms that increase public awareness of critical children issues.

All of these services are essential components of HIV/AIDS education. Public schools need not couch their AIDS education and prevention programs on formal instructional modules; students need more than formal instructions about HIV and AIDS. Although schools are agents for achieving the health objectives for the nation, not all AIDS and HIV education programs are equal; they vary in quality. If schools can build coalitions with CBOs, it would improve teachers' understanding of AIDS, the dissemination of information about AIDS, and the implementation of education and prevention programs for three distinct populations: the general student population, students at risk for HIV infection, and students with HIV or AIDS. Additionally, schools must be reminded that some of these services are sometimes free or inexpensive. Therefore, public schools should take advantage of the community resources available to them. For now, AIDS prevention is only possible through education that effects behavioral change. Community-based organizations can help public schools achieve this objective.

References

"AIDS in 13–24 Age Range Grows 62% in Two Years" (1992, April 11). *Los Angeles Times,* p. A-14.

Alali, A. O. (1992). *Fear of AIDS as a Media Construct.* Unpublished manuscript.

Bailey, M. E. (1991, November-December). "Community-Based Organizations and CDC as Partners in HIV Education and Prevention." *Public Health Reports,* 106(6):702–708.

Center for Population Options (1989, March 31). *Partnership Program.* (Center for Population Options Annual Report, 1988–1989). Washington, DC: CPO.

____ (1983). *Sexuality Education Strategy and Resource Guide: Peer Education Programs.* Washington, DC: CPO.

Forrest, J. D., and Silverman, J. (1989, March-April). "What Public School Teachers Teach About Preventing Pregnancy, AIDS and Sexually Transmitted Diseases." *Family Planning Perspectives,* 21(2):65–72.

Haffner, D. W. (1987, November). *AIDS and Adolescents: The Time for Prevention Is Now.* Washington, DC: Center for Population Options.

____ (1994, August/September). "The Good News About Sexuality Education, 1994." *SIECUS Report,* 22(6):17–18.

Hugick, L., and Leonard, J. (1991, October). "Sex in America." *Gallup Poll Monthly,* 313:60–73.

Kantor, L. (1994, February-March). "Who Decides? Parents and Comprehensive Sexuality Education." *SIECUS Report,* 22(3):7–13.

National Broadcasting Corporation (1987, January 16). *NBC News Poll Results.* New York: NBC.

Schmiedeskamp, J. (1991, November). "Magic Johnson's AIDS Announcement Has Dramatic Impact on Young People." *Gallup Poll Monthly,* 314:2–4.

Shayne, V. T., and Kaplan, B. J. (1988, December). "AIDS Education for Adolescents." *Youth & Society,* 20(2):180–208.

Chapter Twelve

Criteria for Evaluating an AIDS Curriculum

NATIONAL COALITION
OF ADVOCATES FOR STUDENTS

When five people met in early 1987 to draft the first edition of *Criteria for Evaluating an AIDS Curriculum,* school staff around the country were just beginning to realize that they had a responsibility to include HIV education in the school program. At the time, few teachers and administrators knew enough about the epidemic to choose from among the AIDS curricula then appearing on the market. This booklet was developed to guide them in making those choices.

The shifting patterns of the epidemic that were just becoming apparent in 1987 are now disturbingly clear. The virus has taken root in our nation's adolescent population. Between January 1990 and January 1992, the number of United States teenagers diagnosed with AIDS increased by 171 percent. A disproportionate number of these adolescents are African-American or Latino. The epidemic has now spread far beyond a few urban epicenters. In fact, between 1989 and 1990, diagnosed cases of AIDS in rural areas increased by 37 percent, compared to a 5 percent increase in metropolitan areas. As HIV infection spreads further into the American population, the percentage of cases acquired by heterosexual contact also increases.

As of March 1992, 32 states (and the District of Columbia) have mandated that HIV education be included in the school curriculum. Paralleling this increased commitment to educating school-age youth about HIV is an ever greater array of educational materials. Some, in NCAS' opinion, are educationally sound and medically accurate; others are confusing, incomplete, and ineffective; still others are inaccurate, biased, and potentially harmful.

This chapter presents a set of criteria that can be used to evaluate and compare HIV curricula. It includes developmental characteristics of students at different grade levels and appropriate approaches to HIV education in those grades. An effective staff training program and strategies for parent and community involvement are also outlined. Since 1987, school administrators and teachers have used it to select HIV education materials. Curriculum developers have used its guidelines in writing new curricula. Parents have used it to advocate for quality HIV education programs for their children. National, state, and local organizations, as well as individual trainers have included it in numerous policy manuals and HIV training packets. This is our second revision.

Since its first draft, *Criteria* has been a work in progress. It has been fine-tuned, then fine-tuned again. It reflects the input of numerous educators, parents, child development experts, representatives of communities of color, advocates, and youth.

This newest revision further fine-tunes the document. While most changes highlight themes present from earlier versions, the points of increased emphasis are subtle, but important:

- HIV education should take place in the context of a larger program of comprehensive school health education.
- Peer education is an important component of HIV education.
- All youth, both gay and straight, need accurate information delivered in a straightforward, nonjudgmental way.
- HIV infection should be presented as a spectrum of disease.
- Adolescents have special needs in relation to HIV test counseling and support.

We hope you will find *Criteria* helpful in setting standards for an HIV education program that equips students with accurate information, then teaches them the necessary skills to make healthy decisions.

Basic Criteria

Adolescents and young adults are at risk for infection with the human immunodeficiency virus (HIV) that causes acquired immunodeficiency syndrome (AIDS). At least 50 percent of all teenagers are sexually active; most will have more than one sexual partner, and some teenagers will experiment with drugs. Regardless of whether adults approve of these behaviors, young people's lives are at risk. Schools must assume a key role in teaching youth the information and skills they need to avoid contracting this deadly disease.

Instruction about HIV, AIDS, and other sexually transmitted diseases (STDs) should take place within a K–12 comprehensive health education program that establishes a foundation for understanding the relationship between health and behavior. Such a program should address sexuality, injury prevention, drug and alcohol abuse, exercise, nutrition, and tobacco use, in addition to HIV and AIDS. Each component of such a sequential course of study should reinforce decision making, assertiveness, and communication skills learned in previous units.

The goal of health education must be to help students adopt healthy behaviors. A skill-based approach is critical because knowledge alone is insufficient. The HIV component should present the positive aspects of sexuality as well as the risks. It must be appropriate to the chronological and developmental age of the student as is suggested in the section "Matching Approaches" and should be taught in groups of 20 or fewer students.

The following checklist can assist parents, child advocates, school board members, teachers, and administrators in evaluating existing HIV curricula and in advocating for the establishment of high quality HIV education programs.

Curriculum Content An effective HIV curriculum should elicit "yes" answers to these questions:

- Does the curriculum allay young children's unwarranted fears of AIDS?
- Does the curriculum give young children a foundation for a more detailed discussion of sexuality and health at the fifth grade level and later?
- For students in grades six and higher, does the curriculum give simple, clear, and direct information about HIV transmission and prevention? (See section on "What adolescents should know about AIDS and HIV, p. 138.")
- By identifying high-risk behaviors rather than high-risk groups, does the curriculum strongly convey the message that *anyone* who engages in risk behaviors can become infected with HIV regardless of race, gender, age, or sexual orientation?
- Does the curriculum focus on teaching students how to make healthy decisions about sex and drug use and not on simply providing information about the medical aspects of HIV and AIDS?
- Does the curriculum present the material in a manner that does not judge or preach?
- Does the curriculum affirm that it is natural for people to have sexual feelings?
- Are students taught how to assess their own personal risk of HIV infection?
- Does the curriculum help students acquire the necessary self-esteem and assertiveness to choose to abstain from sexual intercourse?
- Does the curriculum inform all students about effective ways to prevent infection if they become sexually active, including information about condoms, their correct use, ways to obtain them, and how to discuss condom use with sexual partners?
- Does the curriculum discuss same-gender as well as opposite gender sexual activity in a straightforward, nonjudgmental way?

- Do any pictures or stories reflect people of different races and ethnic groups? Do they reflect different types of family configurations?
- Are several class periods provided to give students multiple opportunities to rehearse making healthy decisions about risk behaviors based on the information they have learned about AIDS and other STDs?

Development and Implementation

- Is the curriculum updated regularly to incorporate new information as it becomes available?
- Does the curriculum involve students in the HIV education of their peers?
- Does the program provide for adequate staff training to teach the curriculum? (See section on "Staff Training," p. 140.)
- Are staff members helped to examine their own attitudes about sexuality and AIDS?
- Are staff members given accurate and detailed information about HIV and other STDs?
- Are staff members taught the necessary skills to teach an HIV curriculum effectively?
- Is the same information given to students with limited English proficiency in their own language?
- Is an appropriate teaching strategy used to educate students with healing and visual impairments and students with severely disabling conditions?
- Are materials written on a reading level appropriate to the students in the class?
- Do teachers have the necessary backing of parents and administrators to teach sensitive material in a direct manner?
- Have specific school policies been established to support HIV education?
- Has sufficient community and parental support been generated?
- Does the curriculum facilitate an ongoing dialogue with parents on these issues? (See section on "Parental and Community Involvement," p. 142.)

Matching Approaches to HIV Education with Childhood Development

An effective HIV education program will be developmentally based. Very young children do not understand cause or prevention. They need their fears allayed. Fourth and fifth graders can understand causes and "non-causes" of disease but are generally too young to understand how certain behaviors cause disease. Instruction can focus on identifying and differentiating what does and does not cause AIDS. By sixth or seventh grade, however, students can begin to understand illness as a syndrome and how specific causes result in HIV infection. Prevention must be emphasized at this level.

Students in particular grade will vary widely in their emotional, physical, and cognitive development. Teachers are urged to individualize their teaching where appropriate, while keeping in mind that the following statements may characterize the majority of their students.

Grades K Through Three Students are likely:

- to be egocentric; that is, to view the world from their own perspective, making little decision between their own points of view and those of others;
- to develop some independence from parents and gradually to orient toward peers;
- to be curious about external body parts;
- to be highly competitive and capable of unkindness to each other;
- to understand information in terms of their own experiences;
- to perceive cause and effect in terms of mere happenstance;
- to trust the information given to them by authority figures;
- not to understand the sexual terms and events they discuss.

Grades Four and Five Students are likely to be:

- in different stages of prepuberty and early puberty;
- becoming aware of sexual feelings and desires—either in themselves or in others—and confused about them;
- increasingly sensitive to peer pressure;
- capable of concern for others;
- exploring sex roles;
- interested in learning about sexuality and human relationships;
- able to discuss human sexuality;
- still confused between what really is and what might be possible;
- able to internalize rules and know what is right or wrong according to those rules;
- able to perceive only linear, unidirectional, cause-effect relationships;
- interested in discrete lists of causes and "non-causes" of illnesses;
- interested in internal body parts; perceiving the body as a collection of discrete parts;
- focused on concrete aspects of body parts, such as size, color, and shape.

Grades Six Through Nine Students are likely to be:

- engaged in a search for identity (including sexual identity);
- asking "Who am I?" and "Am I normal?";
- very centered on self;

- influenced by peer attitudes;
- concerned about and experimenting with relationships between boys and girls;
- confused about the range of heterosexual and homosexual feelings many of them will have experienced;
- worried about the changes in their bodies;
- interested in internal body functioning and able to view body as an integrated system;
- able to understand that behavior has consequences, but perhaps not to believe that the consequences could happen to them;
- fearful of asking questions about sex that might make them appear uninformed;
- beginning to understand complex relationships between multiple causes and multiple effects with regard to illness; that is, to understand the concept of "interaction";
- beginning to understand the notion of prevention.

Grades Ten Through Twelve Students are likely to be:

- still struggling for a sense of personal identity, especially those students who are confused about their sexual identities;
- thinking that they "know it all";
- seeking greater independence from parents;
- still heavily influenced by peers, but open to information provided by trusted adults;
- near the end of this period, beginning to think about establishing more permanent relationships;
- experiencing a sense of denial about their vulnerability to AIDS and other dangers;
- sexually active.

Appropriate Approaches to HIV Education

Grades K Through Three The primary goal at this level is to allay children's unwarranted fears of AIDS and to establish a foundation for understanding the relationship between health and behavior.

- Information about AIDS and HIV should be included in the larger curriculum on body appreciation, wellness, sickness, friendships, assertiveness, family roles, and different types of families.
- Children should be encouraged to feel positively about their bodies and to know their external body parts and the differences between girls and boys. Teachers should answer their questions about how babies are conceived, born, and how they develop.

- AIDS should be defined simply as a very serious disease that afflicts some adults and teenagers. Students should be told that young children rarely have AIDS and that they do not need to worry about playing with children whose parents have AIDS or with those few children with the disease. They should be reassured that scientists are working hard to find a cure.
- Children should be cautioned never to play with hypodermic syringes or needles found on playgrounds or elsewhere and to avoid contact with other people's blood.
- Questions should be answered directly and simply; responses should be limited to questions asked.
- Children should be taught assertiveness about refusing unwanted touch by others, including family members.
- Children should be told that not all people who "have sex" or "do drugs" get AIDS.

Grades Four and Five The same approach is appropriate for this level as that used for grades K–3. Increased emphasis, however, should be placed on certain points.

- Children should be reassured that it is natural to have sexual feelings.
- Children may need help examining and affirming their own and their families' values.
- Basic information should be provided about human sexuality, disease prevention, healthy choices, functions of the body, and the changes that occur during puberty. Teachers should not assume that children who use sexually explicit language understand what they are saying.
- Basic information should be provided about what does and does not cause AIDS.

Grades Six Through Twelve The primary goal at this level is to teach students to protect themselves and others from infection with HIV and other STDs.

- Students should be taught all of the information in the section on "What Adolescents Should Know About AIDS and HIV."
- The threat of HIV infection and AIDS should be made as real as possible without overly frightening the students. Movies about AIDS or classroom visits from people with AIDS or HIV infection have helped students in some schools understand that HIV is a real threat that they must face. People with AIDS give a human face to lessons about the disease.
- Instruction should be focused on healthy behaviors rather than on the medical aspects of the disease.
- Students should be encouraged to examine and affirm their own values.
- Students should be assured that they have a right to abstain from sexual

intercourse or to postpone becoming sexually active. They should be helped to develop the skills to assert this right.

- Students should rehearse making responsible decisions about sex and drug use, including responses to risky behavioral situations.
- An effective program will teach students how to evaluate reasonable and unreasonable risk while acknowledging that some types of experimentation are a healthy aspect of adolescent development.
- Teachers must not assume that all students will choose abstinence.
- Teachers must not assume that all students are sexually active.
- Students should be taught in a matter-of-fact, nonjudgmental manner how to use a condom and where to buy or obtain one. They should be encouraged to hold and unroll a condom. All students, whether or not they are sexually active, should be taught that condoms are an essential protection from HIV for all types of sexual intercourse.
- Students should be helped to recognize that affection and intimacy can be expressed in ways other than sexual intercourse.
- Students who are sexually active should be encouraged to reduce their risk of HIV infection by identifying sexual activities which do not involve intercourse.
- Information about HIV should be presented along with information about other STDs and drug use.
- It is important to be honest and to provide information in a straightforward manner. Be explicit. Use simple, clear words. Explain in detail. Use examples.
- Sexual terms must be clearly defined.
- Teachers should be non-threatening and work to alleviate anxiety among students.
- Students should be given the opportunity to ask questions anonymously.
- Discussion of dating relationships can provide opportunities to teach decision-making skills. Students should be helped to think through how to make responsible decisions about sex before questions arise in a dating context.
- Teaching about AIDS and HIV is often enhanced by videos and other visual aids; role plays and other participatory exercises; same-sex groupings (to encourage more candid discussion) followed by sharing in a mixed-sex group (to increase comfort level in discussing sexual subjects with members of the opposite sex); and involvement of students in planning and teaching—letting young people speak the message to each other whenever possible.
- HIV education should also include discussion of critical social issues raised by the epidemic, such as weighing the protection of the public health against endangering individual liberties and the impact of the HIV epidemic on the health care system.

- Teachers should help students find answers to detailed medical questions.

What Adolescents Should Know About AIDS and HIV

Adolescents need information about AIDS and HIV that is simple and straightforward. Home and school instruction should emphasize prevention by teaching safe behaviors. Although adolescents need only minimal knowledge of the medical aspects of the disease, some of them may seek a more in-depth understanding of the virus and its manifestations. Teachers and parents should be prepared to answer their questions.

The following information should be appropriately communicated to all adolescents.

Definitions of HIV and AIDS Acquired immunodeficiency syndrome is an infectious disease caused by infection with the human immunodeficiency virus (HIV). The virus usually weakens the immune system, making the infected person vulnerable to certain diseases that healthy people can fight off, but that can be fatal to a person with AIDS. Unlike most infections, HIV infection cannot be eliminated. The virus remains in the person's body for the rest of her or his life.

Transmission of HIV The virus is transmitted in three ways:

1. through infected semen and vaginal secretions—by vaginal or anal sexual intercourse or by oral sex;
2. through infected blood—by sharing hypodermic needles or syringes for injecting illegal drugs or by using unsterile needles or syringes for taking steroids, vitamins, antibiotics, for skin popping, piercing ears, tattooing, or any other purpose;
3. from an infected woman to her child either before or during childbirth or through breast milk.

Anyone who engages in risky behaviors with an infected person can become infected, regardless of gender, sexual orientation, age, or race.

HIV is not transmitted by casual contact such as hugging, sneezing, or sharing bathrooms.

A person does not become infected with HIV by donating blood. Several years ago, some people became infected through receiving blood transfusions. Today, however, all blood donations in the U.S. are screened and tested so that there is little risk of HIV infection through blood transfusions.

Sexually Transmitted Diseases Unprotected sexual intercourse can result in other sexually transmitted infections besides HIV. These other infections can seriously affect a person's health and are much more common than HIV infection. Most STDs can be easily treated.

Spectrum of HIV Infection Many people infected with HIV go through long periods when they have no symptoms of disease. Since they look and feel healthy, these people may not know they are infected. They can, however, transmit the virus to others through unprotected sexual intercourse, sharing unsterile needles or syringes, or childbirth or breast-feeding.

Persons infected with HIV will develop over time symptoms of a damaged immune system. They may be only mildly ill or very sick. They may remain free from symptoms for 10 years or more.

An advanced stage of HIV infection is AIDS. Someone diagnosed with AIDS becomes sick with infections and cancers that people with healthy immune systems can fight off. People with HIV disease can also exhibit neurological problems.

Testing for HIV Infection A blood test can determine, in almost all cases, whether or not a person has been infected with HIV. This is not a test for AIDS, but rather a test for antibodies to HIV.

Students who engage in behaviors that place them at risk for HIV infection should be advised to consider testing to determine whether they are infected. Life-prolonging treatment is now available for people in early stages of HIV disease.

Any student, however, who considers HIV antibody testing faces complex psychological and legal issues. Few test sites have counselors with experience in the special issues of adolescents at risk for HIV infection. Pretest and posttest counseling available to adults may not be adequate for adolescents.

Counseling and support services must be available to any student who considers testing. This counseling must be comprehensive; culturally specific in the student's own language; geared to the student's cognitive abilities, psychological needs, and sexual orientation; and offered in a safe environment.

Students must understand the difference between HIV infection and having AIDS, anonymous and confidential test sites, and false-negative and false-positive test results, as well as the importance of adopting risk-reduction behaviors regardless of the test results. Students must also understand that a person may not develop antibodies to HIV for six months after infection.

It is recommended that adolescents be tested in a site where ongoing follow-up medical and mental health care is available, such as an adolescent clinic, community health center, or family planning clinic. The confidentiality of an adolescent considering or moving ahead with testing should be strictly guaranteed. Although not always statutorily explicit, legal authority exists in almost all states for physicians to test mature and competent adolescents without parental consent.

Students should be referred to a source of skilled counseling on adolescent testing issues rather than referred directly for testing. Comprehensive posttest counseling and medical follow-up must also be provided, including the identification of responsible adult support.

Avoiding Infection Adolescents can prevent infection with HIV by:

- abstaining from or postponing sexual activity.
- having sexual relations only within the context of a mutually faithful relationship with an uninfected partner.
- always using latex condoms (even in combination with other forms of birth control) from erection to withdrawal of penis and for all types of intercourse. When using a condom, one should use only water-based lubricants. If used properly, latex condoms are very effective in preventing HIV transmission.
- not using intravenous drugs. Those who do should be encouraged to enter a drug treatment program. Those who continue to use drugs should never share needles or syringes, but if they do, they should be told how to sterilize their equipment. Tattoo needles and needles used for injecting vitamins, antibiotics, body-building hormones, or piercing ears should never be shared.

Treatment and Cure There is neither a cure for HIV infection nor a vaccine to prevent it. An increasing number of treatments, however, are proving effective in prolonging life and, if administered early enough, in delaying the onset of symptoms.

Local Telephone Numbers Students should be given a local telephone number to call for additional information. Sources of AIDS and HIV information in other languages should also be provided. Some local AIDS hotlines have Spanish-speaking staff available during certain hours. Find out what these hours are and provide this information to Spanish-speaking students. Health clinics and other community organizations serving Latino, Southeast Asian, and other non–English-speaking communities may also be able to provide HIV counseling in their languages.

The following national hotlines can provide information about state and local hotlines and AIDS services:

- 1-800-342-AIDS (AIDS information in English, 24 hours a day)
- 1-800-344-SIDA (AIDS information in Spanish, 8 AM–2 AM EST)
- 1-800-243-7889 (TTY-TDD-AIDS information for hearing-impaired people, M–F 10 AM–10 PM EST)
- 1-800-227-8922 (National Sexually Transmitted Diseases Hotline)

Staff Training

Staff training is a must. The following two levels of training should be provided.

Basic Training in AIDS and HIV Prevention for All School Staff All staff (teachers, administrators, custodians, and clerical personnel) should receive basic information about AIDS and HIV. They should understand its transmission and prevention and should know where in the school and community to get more information and help.

Education on HIV at this level can be conducted as a one- or two-session in-service workshop. Public health departments and local AIDS service agencies can usually provide knowledgeable workshop leaders.

Each school should designate an HIV resource person. A similar HIV resource staff person should be located at the central office level of each school district.

Specialized Training for Teachers of HIV Prevention All teachers and supervisory administrators who will be teaching HIV prevention education should receive more comprehensive training than that given to all school staff. When feasible, participants should be offered graduate-level credit.

Special efforts should be made to recruit and train teachers who share the same racial and cultural backgrounds as large subgroups of the student population.

There are three components of effective training to teach HIV prevention. The first is the establishment of context. Before staff members are trained to teach a curriculum, a supportive environment for the program must be developed within the community. A community public education campaign can help parents and other members of the community understand the importance of HIV prevention education. This understanding will free teachers to discuss with students the many sensitive issues raised by the HIV epidemic. (See section on "Parental and Community Involvement," p. 142.)

The second component is the content of the training. It should include accurate and detailed information about AIDS and HIV presented to the participants in a way that alleviates their own fears of exposure to the virus; an examination of the sensitive and controversial issues involved in HIV prevention; an opportunity for staff to look at their own attitudes about sexuality and AIDS and to recognize that there exists a broad range of views about sexuality; and a workshop on effective ways to address the special needs of gay and lesbian youth; classroom strategies and activities, including models for integrating AIDS and HIV education into comprehensive programs of school health education.

The third component is methodology. Teachers should be trained to instruct students in a way that humanizes the issues and helps students realize that HIV affects them. Training should enable teachers to identify specific student behaviors that they want to influence and skills that students need to affect those behaviors. These skills concern decision making, effective communication, and assertiveness. Teachers should be further trained to provide a context in which students can practice using these skills. A good training program will give teachers practice in building the skills they in turn will teach their students.

Teachers who are uncomfortable with the subject matter should not be required to teach an HIV unit. Their confusion and discomfort inevitably will be conveyed to their students. Teachers who agree to teach HIV units should be offered opportunities to team teach or to draw on outside resource people for support and assistance. Family planning agencies can help identify sexuality educators to lead this training. Effective training may also involve significant participation of parents and students. (This attachment is based, in large part, on training strategies developed by ETR Associates, Santa Cruz, CA.)

Parental and Community Involvement

Parents and community leaders should be included in the development and implementation of HIV curricula. By involving them, you will:

- educate key community members about HIV and AIDS and the risks to adolescents;
- involve parents and community members in an important way in their children's education;
- develop a curriculum that considers the ethnic and cultural roots of sexual attitudes;
- build respect and a broad validation for the curriculum;
- build a solid base of supportive community members;
- give teachers the support they need to teach sensitive material in a direct manner.

HIV Education Advisory Committees An advisory committee can work with key school personnel to design a program, provide information to the community, and present the program to the local school board. The committee might include parents, religious leaders, student leaders, elected officials, and staff members of community agencies. The committee should reflect the true racial and ethnic diversity of the community. Although all members should concur on the importance of effective AIDS and HIV education, committee members should reflect a broad range of community perspectives.

While the primary mandate of the advisory committee is the timely implementation of an HIV curriculum, the committee should also lay the groundwork for a planned and sequential kindergarten through grade 12 comprehensive health education program. In addition to HIV education, this program would address drug, alcohol, and tobacco use; human sexuality; injury control; sexually transmitted diseases; exercise; consumer and environmental education; and nutrition. Through such a comprehensive program, students can acquire the self-esteem and decision-making skills necessary to make healthy choices about HIV and other important life issues.

A Parental Component of the HIV Curriculum At the same time students are being taught about HIV, parents should also be educated about the disease, its transmission, and its prevention. A well-planned and publicized information night for parents is one method. A second effective strategy is a parent-student communication component built into the curriculum itself. Students are then empowered to be educators themselves, perhaps assisted by a study guide to use in teaching their parents. This approach will reinforce classroom learning, educate parents about AIDS and HIV, and facilitate a dialogue between students and parents about sexuality issues.

A Collaborative Community and School HIV Prevention Initiative Pilot projects for adolescent pregnancy prevention in several communities across the country have demonstrated good results when schools, churches, local media agencies, health institutions, and youth-serving community groups mount a simultaneous organized, and complementary health education and services campaign. These outcomes indicate that school-based HIV education is more likely to affect student behavior when it is part of a coordinated, community-wide campaign.

Chapter Thirteen

Selecting and Evaluating Audiovisuals for an AIDS/HIV Education

A. ODASUO ALALI

The literature related to public health communication campaigns seems to demonstrate persuasively that the mass media are effective in disseminating adequate and accurate information about serious health problems and in increasing public awareness about diseases (Arkin, 1990). Although this may well be the case, the proliferation of media technology and the expansion of instruments of communication have presented public health educators with difficult choices. As Kreps (1988) observes, "The role of communication and information in health care is so ubiquitous, equivocal, and pervasive that it is often taken for granted and complexities and subtleties of health communication are often unnoticed, incompletely analyzed, and ineffectively used."

The acquired immunodeficiency syndrome (AIDS) epidemic has not diminished the seriousness of this problem. In essence, public health educators are still faced with the difficult choices of selecting appropriate media campaigns for AIDS education and prevention. In some cases, this problem has been "resolved," as public health educators use whatever media campaign is available to them without the benefit of practical, valid, dependable guidelines for making those choices (Campeau, 1974). In other cases, their choices are influenced by what they already know about mass media's role in health-related issues, such as the tobacco control programs (Bauman et al., 1988; Flay, 1987) and the campaign to reduce cardiovascular disease (Bellicha & McGrath, 1990). Additionally, in his review of the uses of audiovisuals in instruction, Campeau (1974) argues that "all indications are that decisions as to which audiovisual devices to purchase, install, and use have been based on administering and organizational requirements and on consideration of costs, availability, and user preference, not on evidence of instructional effectiveness."

Although such decisions as Campeau mentions rests on a sound knowledge base, common-sense methods of decision making are neither adequate nor particularly useful in the selection and evaluation of audiovisuals for public health campaigns, especially in AIDS education and prevention. Each public health problem requires a separate education and prevention approach, and AIDS is a unique disease that requires a specific approach aimed at behavior change. Its uniqueness is defined by who gets AIDS and how the general public reacts to these individuals. Overall, the disease has elicited intense emotional reaction in those who are not infected with regard to those who are. The result has been fear (or "AFRAIDS") that has created myths and misperceptions about the disease. Therefore, the selection and evaluation of audiovisuals for AIDS education and prevention should consider these issues, as well as the cultural variables that encourage denial in at-risk populations and the personal factors that differ among various at-risk groups. In essence, decisions in selecting audiovisuals should be based on their instructional effectiveness.

Before selecting audiovisuals and evaluating their instructional effectiveness, specific variables must be considered. The selection should be done carefully, especially at public schools. The AIDS epidemic has spawned a plethora of audiovisual materials, some of which are inadequate for AIDS education and prevention (Sawyer & Beck, 1991, p. 32). Clearly, this illustrates the concern and need for specific guidelines that will facilitate the selection and evaluation process.

Why Are Audiovisuals Important in AIDS Education?

Historically, audiovisual media (e.g., film strips, still photographs, slides, motion pictures, disc recordings, audiotape recordings, videotape recordings, and transparencies) have been used in educational settings to augment formal instructions. Just as audiovisuals have had a profound effect on traditional education, they are likely to be catalysts in AIDS education and prevention in public schools.

Reasons why audiovisuals should be used in AIDS education and prevention in public schools include the following:

1. Audiovisuals can be tools for providing adequate and accurate information about AIDS.
2. Audiovisuals can reflect the diverse ethnic and cultural groups in the target population.
3. Audiovisual contents are easily previewed for reaction and feedback before acquisition.

4. Audiovisual information can easily be directed at the specific health needs of a group.

5. Audiovisuals encourage on-the-spot interaction with students.

6. Audiovisuals are individual and personal media that provide intimate methods of learning and encourage viewers to take responsibility for their health.

7. Audiovisuals can be applied to group learning situations.

8. Audiovisuals are inexpensive. They can be purchased or rented at a relatively low price.

9. The auditory and visual codes in audiovisual presentations facilitate the recognition, retention, and recall of messages.

10. Audiovisuals can reinforce and construct intended meaning for the viewer. The degree of persuasiveness depends, however, on the quality of the audiovisual.

11. The Centers for Disease Control (CDC) recognize the potential of audiovisual media in AIDS education and prevention (CDC, 1990). Nonprofit organizations and community-based groups also use AIDS-related audiovisuals.

12. There are numerous AIDS education and prevention audiovisuals to choose from.

Guidelines for Selecting Audiovisual Media

In a review of the effects of videotapes on perceived susceptibility to HIV and AIDS among university freshmen, Sawyer and Beck (1991) argue that although audiovisual materials are commonplace today, "little objective evaluation has been performed" (p. 32). This study echoes the findings of previous research that has obligated researchers to develop guidelines that schools and public health educators can use to select and evaluate audiovisual devices. In such one study, Campeau (1974) observes that "to date, media research in post-school education has not provided decision makers with practical, valid, dependable guidelines for making choices on the basis of instructional effectiveness."

Instructional effectiveness becomes crucial when one considers that numerous organizations have produced thousands of audiovisuals, some of which provide little factual knowledge about AIDS (Gilliam & Seltzer, 1989; Rhodes & Wolitski, 1989). This plethora of audiovisuals can serve, if selections are not made carefully, to collaborate in the miseducation of students, which in turn has negative effects on AIDS education and prevention.

In order to facilitate the selection and evaluation of audiovisuals for AIDS education and prevention in public schools, the following guidelines are recommended.

Message Objective The selection and evaluation of audiovisuals should be based on specific message objectives. The CDC identifies three principal components to HIV education and prevention strategies: public information and education, education for school-age populations, and risk reduction (including counseling and testing of high-risk individuals). Although the CDC guidelines specify these goals for any HIV education and prevention program, they also leave room for expansion. To these guidelines, one may add specific elements that address not only factual information, but the myths and misperceptions associated with HIV.

Consequently, quality audiovisuals should have the attributes that not only inform, educate, or provide counseling and referrals for the target audience, but also incorporate decision making and communication skills that are of value to the specific population. Questions to consider regarding the message objectives when evaluating and selecting audiovisual media include the following:

1. Does the audiovisual define AIDS? How?
2. Does the audiovisual teach that AIDS is an infectious disease caused by a virus and that it leads to death?
3. Does it emphasize the need to practice safer behaviors, and are these explained?
4. Does the audiovisual deal with other methods of preventing HIV infection or transmission?
5. Does the audiovisual deal with the effectiveness of each prevention method?
6. Does the audiovisual refute common myths, misperceptions, and misinformation about AIDS?
7. Does the audiovisual try to reduce anxiety and fear?
8. Does it emphasize risk behaviors rather than risk groups?
9. Does it provide information about counseling and referrals?
10. Does the audiovisual show that AIDS is not a gay disease?
11. Does the audiovisual emphasize that decision making and communication with one's partner are important ways to prevent infection?
12. What specific themes are used to encourage prevention?
13. Does the audiovisual examine the relationship between knowledge and behavior?

Modes of Transmission Another key element in evaluating and selecting audiovisual media for AIDS education and prevention is whether the modes of HIV transmission are addressed. Although audiovisuals should avoid clinical information about disease pathology, it is useful for educational materials to address the ways that HIV is transmitted: sexual contact, contact with infected blood, sharing of needles by IV drug users, and between mother and fetus or infant.

Following are questions to consider when selecting and evaluating audiovisual materials:

1. Does the audiovisual show how someone can get HIV? What transmission methods are shown?

2. Does the audiovisual show that a person with the AIDS virus can pass it on to someone else through sexual contact?

3. Does the audiovisual indicate that a pregnant woman who has the AIDS virus can give it to her baby?

4. Does the audiovisual show that a person can get HIV by sharing needles for drug use with someone who has the AIDS virus?

5. Does the audiovisual show that one cannot get HIV through casual contact with someone who has the AIDS virus?

Content When evaluating the educational quality of audiovisual materials, experts agree that the content is an important ingredient that measures how effective the presentation will be. One can draw support from Wilbur Schramm's (1977) analysis of the media, which argues that "over and over again the answer has come back: of course, students can learn effectively from the media, from any medium. It depends on the performance of the teacher, the content of the media, what is being taught, and to whom" (p. 14).

Suter and Waddell (1981), after reviewing the attributes of quality in audiovisuals in health education, conclude that "the ultimate test for quality of educational material is a measure of their impact on learning and behavior" (p. 5). Education and prevention programs in HIV and AIDS are consistently tested by the amount of knowledge they provide and whether such information results in behavior change. Audiovisuals used in HIV education should be appropriate tools that withstand this test.

Content is a measure of appropriateness. Therefore, to determine whether an audiovisual is appropriate for the specific AIDS education, its content should be indexed by the following ten questions:

1. Is the information accurate, relevant, and up-to-date?
2. Is the information appropriate for the target audience?
3. Is the information simple and not confusing for the educational level of the target audience?
4. Does the audiovisual avoid medical jargon and confusing statistics?
5. Is the information objective and devoid of bias?
6. Can the information motivate learning in the target audience?
7. Is the information appropriate to the target audience's situation?
8. Is the information authoritative and supported by scientific evidence?
9. Is the information free of all controversial religious, political, or ideological views? If not, are these controversies addressed?
10. Can learning be accomplished in the amount of time spent using the audiovisual material?

Visual and Auditory Codes The use of audiovisuals offers students an alternative learning experience that enhances their understanding of the subject matter. Additionally, visual and auditory presentations have been found to generate interest among students, as well as to serve as persuasive tools for behavioral change. Clearly, audiovisual presentations are memorable to students because they most likely are appropriate to the viewer's situation.

Audiovisuals for AIDS education are not as easy to select and evaluate as they are to find: "Technical advances of recent years have led to an increasing armamentarium of educational resources at the disposal of instructors and students" (Suter & Waddell, 1981, p. 5). With this plethora of resources comes information overload, or what Stein (1979, p. 23) calls "mediaitis." In offering a sweeping guideline on selecting and evaluating media for patient education, Stein suggests that "an overdose and prolonged exposure to inappropriate visual and auditory stimulations" (p. 23) could lead to mediaitis. This is to say that inappropriate visual and auditory codes usually affect the meaning of the message. Therefore, visual and auditory codes are important considerations in the transmission of messages.

The following are questions that should guide AIDS educators' evaluation of appropriate visual and auditory codes of audiovisual media:

1. Do the visuals communicate the story and situation clearly?
2. Are the visuals of any educational significance to the target audience?
3. Are the visual representations aesthetically pleasing (lighting, color, tone, contrast, etc.)?
4. Are informational graphics used? If so, are they appropriate to the viewer situation?
5. Do the visuals compete with auditory elements, or complement them? If the former, how effective is the audiovisual as a learning tool?
6. Are the voices in the audiovisual clear?
7. Can a viewer identify with the visual illustrations used?
8. Are inappropriate visual and auditory codes used?
9. Are the performers believable?
10. Do viewers identify with the performers?

Target Audience The term target audience describes a specific public served by a medium. This concept is of import to public health campaigns because it helps to define the specific audience that campaigners must impress. In other words, a target audience defines the ways a public health educator should design, conduct, and implement a campaign. From an AIDS education perspective, one can argue that the nature of the target audience defines the nature of the campaign.

The challenges posed by different audiences, as well as different approaches and perspectives, require that appropriate guidelines be used to conceptualize the public health audience and to determine campaign audiovisuals. Questions that define the quality of an audiovisual relative to its target audience include the following:

1. Does the audiovisual define its intended public?
2. Does the audiovisual identify the relevant categories of at-risk populations for HIV infection?
3. Does the audiovisual identify personal characteristics, values, ideologies, and other beliefs that are likely to increase the target audience's chances of HIV infection?
4. Does the audiovisual accommodate the target audience's likely previous experiences?
5. Does the audiovisual link past and future behavior with susceptibility to HIV?
6. Are these messages integrated into the relevant cultures of the target audience?
7. Does the audiovisual recognize each member of the audience as an individual with specific needs?
8. Can learning be self-paced?
9. Does the audiovisual material use a succession of individual experiences to illustrate its points?
10. Does the audiovisual confront the individual's perceived susceptibility to AIDS?
11. Does the audiovisual motivate the target audience not to engage in risky behavior?

Small Group Most young people, particularly adolescents, tend to identify more with their peers than with any other individuals. Because groups are composed of a small number of people (society of friends), they often have a tremendous amount of impact on the attitudes, values, opinions, and behaviors of those who are part of the group. And because most learning at an early age is done in groups (classroom setting), each audiovisual selected for AIDS education and prevention should be flexible for use in both individual and small group settings. Clearly, open discussions, interactions, and shared experiences in group settings do ignite curiosity and interests that, when resolved, could reduce risky behavior.

Questions asked in evaluating this element are as follows:

1. Is the audiovisual adaptable to small group workshops or learning?
2. Is the learning self-paced by the individual, or does it accommodate group teaching?

3. Does the audiovisual give room for topics that can be developed into group discussions?
4. Does the audiovisual encourage collaborative learning?

Feedback Another element in evaluating and selecting audiovisuals for HIV/AIDS education and prevention is determining whether a given audiovisual provides the viewer with opportunity for interaction or seeking additional information. Participation in this educational process can be enhanced by the responses the viewer receives from the audiovisual material.

The criteria for evaluating the effectiveness of an audiovisual for feedback are as follows:

1. Does the audiovisual provide the viewer with a feedback mechanism?
2. Does the audiovisual provide the viewer with information about counseling and referrals?
3. Does the audiovisual direct the viewer to available resources? Where does it say someone can get help to be tested for HIV?
4. Does the audiovisual provide a toll-free telephone number for those seeking additional information?
5. Does the audiovisual provide specific answers to the viewer's questions? Are questions answered instantly?
6. Can the audiovisual be stopped by the instructor at specific intervals to solicit feedback?

Language Version The educational background of the target audience is an important variable that should be considered in evaluating and selecting audiovisual media for HIV education and prevention. At an early stage of life, most students' language and communication skills are not yet fully developed. They must overcome this obstacle in order to understand public health campaigns. The prerequisite for health campaign audiovisuals is whether or not the language of instruction accommodates the different nationalities within the target group. When applying this guideline in the selection of audiovisuals, health educators should be reminded of what Hippocrates said about language: "The chief virtue that language can have is clearness; nothing detracts from it so much as the use of an unfamiliar word."

The appropriateness of an audiovisual in terms of language should be determined by the following questions:

1. Is the audiovisual message presented in the language of the target audience?
2. Are the linguistic versions complex and confusing for the target audience?
3. Is medical jargon avoided?

Ethnic and Cultural Appeal Evaluating and selecting audiovisual media also requires that ethnic and cultural sensitivities be balanced. In an extensive review of visual media for health educators, Lazes and Snyder (1977) found that "most videotapes, films, slides/tape loops were not directed toward diverse cultural and ethnic groups" (p. 4). Clearly, this suggests that the specific ethnic composition and cultural affinity of the target audience be considered in the selection of audiovisual materials for AIDS education and prevention.

An estimate of ethnic and cultural appeal should be indexed by the following questions:

1. Is the audiovisual a culturally appropriate and sensitive tool for AIDS education and prevention?
2. Does the audiovisual accommodate different ethnic populations, specifically ethnic risk groups?
3. Does the audiovisual appeal to different ethnic sensibilities through associations that are culturally identifiable?
4. Does the audiovisual reach out to minority communities?

Corporate Author An important component of this modality is the corporate author of an audiovisual program. There is a relationship between the content of an audiovisual and the producers or sponsors. Appropriate information about the program's origin should be taken into consideration when evaluating and selecting an audiovisual.

Important questions to consider include the following:

1. Are the corporate authors or sponsors identified?
2. Are the corporate authors affiliated with any political or religious organization?
3. Are the corporate authors or sponsors in the regular business of audiovisual production?
4. Are the corporate authors or sponsors recognized as qualified producers of audiovisuals by AIDS specialists and educators?
5. Is information provided about the year of production? Running time?
6. Is the audiovisual catalogued by the Library of Congress?
7. Is the audiovisual widely distributed?
8. Can it be rented or purchased at a reasonable price?
9. Does it provide an instructor's guide?

Clearly, the job of selecting and evaluating audiovisual materials for AIDS education and prevention is a difficult one. It is hoped that these guidelines may help to illuminate the dark alleys public health educators occasionally walk into. They are not to be misconstrued as guarantee that a selected audiovisual will automatically result in the desired behavior change; the persuasiveness of an audiovisual will depend on other personal factors. Regardless, however, one thing is obvious: These guidelines should provide public schools and the health educator with a qualitative and quantitative evaluation mechanism that is of paramount importance to AIDS education and prevention.

References

Arkin, E. B. (1990, May-June). "Opportunities for Improving the Nation's Health Through Collaboration with the Mass Media." *Public Health Reports,* 105(3):219–223.

Bauman, K. E.; Brown, J. D.; Bryan, E. S.; Fisher, L. A.; Padgett, C. A.; and Sweeney, J. M. (1988). "Three Mass Media Campaigns to Prevent Adolescent Cigarette Smoking." *Preventive Medicine,* 17:510–530.

Bellicha, T., and McGrath, J. (1990, May-June). "Mass Media Approaches to Reducing Cardiovascular Disease Risk." *Public Health Reports,* 105(3):245–252.

Campeau, P. L. (1974). "Selective Review of the Results of Research on the Use of Audiovisual Media to Teach Adults." *Audio-Visual Communications Review,* 22: 5–50.

Centers for Disease Control (1990, April). *HIV and AIDS: A Cumulation of the AIDS School Health Education Database.* Atlanta, GA: CDC.

Flay, B. R. (1987, February). "Mass Media and Smoking Cessation: A Critical Review." *American Journal of Public Health,* 77(2):153–160.

Gilliam, A., and Seltzer, R. (1989). "The Efficacy of Educational Movies on AIDS Knowledge and Attitudes Among College Students." *Journal of American College Health,* 37:261–265.

Kreps, G. (1988). "Relational Communication in Health Care." *Southern Speech Communication Journal,* 43:344–359.

Lazes, P. M., and Snyder, D. (1977, July). "Community Oriented Videotapes—Action Tools for Health Educators." *Journal of Biocommunication,* 4(2):4–9.

Rhodes, F., and Wolitski, R. J. (1989). "Effect of Instructional Videotapes on AIDS Knowledge and Attitudes." *Journal of American College Health,* 37:266–271.

Sawyer, R. G., and Beck, K. H. (1991, March-April). "Effects of Videotapes on Perceived Susceptibility to HIV/AIDS Among University Freshmen." *Health Values,* 15(2):31–40.

Schramm, W. (1977). *Big Media, Little Media.* Beverly Hills, CA: Sage Publications.

Stein, D. (1979, November). "Selecting and Evaluating Media for Patient Education." *Journal of Biocommunication,* 6(3):22–26.

Suter, E., and Waddell, W. H. (1981, July). "Attributes of Quality in Audiovisual Material for Health Professionals." *Journal of Biocommunication,* 8(2):5–11.

Chapter Fourteen

Selected Audiovisuals for HIV/AIDS Education

A. ODASUO ALALI
GARY BYRD

Chapter Three provides some evidence of the role mass media play in constructing social reality about acquired immunodeficiency syndrome (AIDS) and those infected with the human immunodeficiency virus (HIV) that causes AIDS. Chapter Thirteen offers a discussion on how the proliferation of media technology and the expansion of the instruments of communication have presented health educators with difficult choices of the appropriate means to disseminate AIDS-related information. Evidence of this difficulty is presented in Kreps's (1988) analysis of rational communication in health care.

More important, the uses of a specific medium (audiovisual) for instructional purposes was reviewed by Campeau (1974), who observes that

> all indications are that decisions as to which audiovisual devices to purchase, install, and use have been based on administering and organizational requirements and on consideration of costs, availability, and user preference, not as evidence of instructional effectiveness.

To help educators rectify this problem, Chapter Thirteen suggests that selection and evaluation of audiovisuals for HIV/AIDS education and prevention should be based on a sound knowledge base that also accommodates the variables that shape individual attitudes and beliefs about a stigmatized disease such as AIDS. Because decisions about audiovisual media must be guided by this perspective, an objective, qualitative evaluation should be performed in the selection of audiovisuals for HIV/AIDS education and prevention.

The purpose of this chapter is to provide educators with a comprehensive list of selected audiovisual media for inclusion in an HIV/AIDS curriculum.

The criteria for selection are based on the guidelines presented in Chapter Thirteen. Although these guidelines alone do not serve as the dominant or determining factors in the selection of the audiovisuals, the following issues reinforce the need for systematic evaluation:

- Most educators tend to be unaware of existing audiovisuals about HIV and AIDS. In some cases, the prescribed curriculum dictates the audiovisuals they use.
- Not all audiovisuals in the market provide accurate and adequate information about HIV and AIDS.
- The audiovisuals presenting facts about the disease may not be appropriate for use at all grade levels. Because of the differences in students' cognitive level at a young age, audiovisual designs about AIDS may be more effective if they are targeted for each grade level.
- Not all audiovisuals stimulate the interactive abilities of students, nor do all of them provide students with the mechanism for feedback. Sometimes interaction-based instructions may help students respond to issues they encounter in their lives. Feedback can also lead to collaborative learning that encourages retention and behavior change.
- Sometimes the cost of audiovisuals is a major concern to educators and affects their choice of audiovisuals. Not all audiovisuals should be purchased; there are rental options.

Supportive Literature

Although the literature on audiovisuals as an instructional tool has not been adequately adjudicated, it has produced supportive evidence that warrants authorizing the use of audiovisual media in HIV/AIDS education and prevention curricula. Sawyer and Beck (1991) investigated the effects of videotapes on the perceived susceptibility of university freshmen to HIV. Although the audiovisuals in their study were not necessarily predictors of safer sex, there appeared to be "a significant increase in perceived susceptibility to HIV in the students who viewed the more effective videotape, particularly in those students who were not yet sexually active." It is likely that students who view audiovisual media messages about HIV increasingly perceive their susceptibility to the virus, thereby becoming more likely to institute safe-sex measures.

Other studies about audiovisual usage in education have produced evidence to suggest their effect on comprehension. One specific example is the research evaluation of a presentation of printed text versus pictorial illustrations (Rohwer & Matz, 1975). The findings suggest that pictorial audiovisual illustrations augment retention of messages. More important is the finding that pictorial presentations are more effective in comprehension recall than are print-related presentations.

Vasu and Howe (1989) provide additional supportive evidence about the effects of visual and verbal modes of presentation on retention. This is confirmed by Nugent (1982), who suggests that the video-print-audio combination is a form of presentation superior to other media forms. Though neither of these studies suggests that knowledge, attitude, and behavior changes may be enhanced by audiovisual messages, there is evidence to support audiovisuals as useful tools for learning. With audiovisuals, students are given the opportunity to experience other instructional modes that stimulate thinking, enhance their intellect, and relate their experiences to the subject matter. By virtue of their visual and auditory modes, and because of their adaptability to cultural variables, audiovisual media can be useful for HIV/AIDS education and prevention curriculum.

Specific Goals for HIV/AIDS Audiovisuals

The principal purpose of AIDS education is to assist students in avoiding infection with the virus that causes the disease. The scope and content of any material used for AIDS education and prevention should be determined by the needs, developmental levels, and cultural backgrounds of the target students. School authorities must realize that it is their responsibility to provide their students with effective school health education, particularly about AIDS: "The nation's public and private schools have the capacity and responsibility to assure that young people understand the nature of the AIDS epidemic and the specific actions they can take to prevent HIV infection" (Centers for Disease Control [CDC], 1988, p. 2).

Although it makes sense that schools should perform their educational responsibilities, existing AIDS/HIV educational programs do not appear to address these concerns. This fact is reflected in an editorial memorandum issued by the Center for Population Options (CPO):

> Existing AIDS and HIV education programs for young people vary greatly in quality. Some integrate information into existing sex education curriculum, emphasizing decision making skills providing exercises that encourage teens to care about themselves and others. Others may approach the topic too narrowly, teaching the bare facts about HIV transmission without providing teens with the motivation and skills to protect themselves. Some programs take the unrealistic "Just Say No" approach to HIV prevention, discussing AIDS as just another terror that preys upon young people who are sexually active [CPO, 1989, pp. 1–2].

Also, because most program and audiovisual selections are haphazardly done, schools must begin to commit their HIV/AIDS curricula to long-term, comprehensive programs. The specific scope and content of AIDS education should be locally determined and should be consistent with the parental and community values where the schools are located.

Where do audiovisuals fit into this equation? Numerous organizations, including the CPO (1988), have suggested specific goals of AIDS education where audiovisuals may fit in. These goals are as follows:

1. To provide accurate information about HIV/AIDS.
2. To eliminate misinformation about the disease.
3. To promote compassion for people with AIDS.
4. To help young people delay the initiation of sexual intercourse.
5. To ensure that young people who are having any type of intercourse use condoms consistently and effectively.
6. To reduce experimentation with drugs, including alcohol, and prevent intravenous (IV) drug use.
7. To help students recognize their personal vulnerability to AIDS.
8. To provide support and counseling services to students.

Method

A search for audiovisuals on HIV/AIDS education was conducted during the months of January, February, and March of 1992. Numerous sources, including the CDC Adolescent School Health database and various audiovisual catalogues, were consulted. The search produced over 100 titles dating from 1988 onwards. A comprehensive content analysis was undertaken to determine their content according to (1) the facts about the disease; (2) knowledge regarding modes of transmission, and personal knowledge about AIDS; (3) attitude (risk perceptions, homophobia, reaction to people with AIDS, and interpersonal AIDS prevention attitudes); and (4) behavior and behavior change.

Accordingly, 27 were selected—some for each of three grade levels (early elementary school, late elementary/middle school, and junior/senior high school) and some for teacher preparation. As much as possible, we present information here that will facilitate the audiovisual adoption process (e.g., telephone number and whether the audiovisual is available for rental or purchase) in the "Audiovisual Ordering Information" section on pages 165 through 167.

Recommended Audiovisuals

Early Elementary School Although educational programs cannot adequately protect a student from infection with HIV, early discussions about the discasc, thc bchaviors that increase infection, and preventive measures are important. The audiovisuals we recommend for this grade level will provide students with the necessary information.

AIDS: Let's Talk. Eugene, OR: New Dimension Media, 1989, 15 minutes.

This program attempts to eliminate unwarranted fears of the AIDS virus held by elementary school children. Positive behaviors are identified instead of name calling and isolating infected children. Also, the program emphasizes that the virus cannot be spread by casual contact and is not transmitted by sneezes, coughs, kisses, toys, drinking glasses, or public bathrooms. The program does not discuss the transmission of the virus by sexual contact. In the process, the program attempts to develop positive attitudes toward other children including those with the AIDS virus. Students are asked to treat persons with AIDS the way they would want to be treated. A handbook accompanies this program.

AIDS: What Every Kid Should Know. Irwindale, CA: Barr Films, n.d., 15 minutes. This engaging, informative film has three learning objectives for elementary students: (1) to describe and define AIDS as a communicable disease; (2) to show how AIDS is and is not contracted; and (3) to show how to prevent contracting AIDS. Additional discussions on myths about contracting AIDS are presented in this program. A brochure accompanies the film.

AIDS and the Immune System. Los Angeles, CA: Churchill Films, 1988, 12 minutes. This program provides elementary school children with the facts about how the human immune system fights disease, and how the AIDS virus attacks the immune system. Additionally, it emphasizes that infection with the AIDS virus is not possible through casual contact, or by sharing food, with an infected child. As an illustration, the video also uses the health condition of two students, one with the flu and the other with the AIDS virus, to show how the flu germ is more contagious by contact than the AIDS virus. The learning objective is for the student to understand that the AIDS virus is transmitted in very limited ways and is difficult to catch.

Ask Me About AIDS. Washington Crossing, PA: Odyssey in Learning, 1988, 14 minutes. The videotape utilizes cartoon characters to present information about the AIDS virus. The program begins with a trio of youngsters opening a book of Greek myths and learning how Zeus gave Pandora a closed box with directions not to open it. Pandora opens the box and lets out a host of evils, which one child suggests may include AIDS. Pandora then asks the children about the AIDS virus and the children respond by telling her what AIDS stands for, how the AIDS virus affects the body's immune system, and that AIDS is a deadly disease for which there is currently no cure or vaccine. They explain to her that AIDS is only spread by the exchange of body fluids, especially blood, and that the exchanges occur only by having sex, by sharing IV drug equipment, by perinatal processes, and occasionally by blood transfusions. The program states that different types of people can get AIDS, including persons who get blood transfusions. The video states that methods of avoiding the AIDS virus include not touching other people's blood or body fluids, not touching needles, and not using drugs. The program concludes by stating that children will not get AIDS if they make the right decisions. A 16-page user's guide accompanies this program.

Beginnings: You Won't Get AIDS. Van Nuys, CA: AIMS Media, 1990, 14 minutes. This program follows the guidelines of the U.S. surgeon general. It provides age-appropriate information about AIDS for children through animated characters, live action and song to try to ease children's fears and answer their questions about how AIDS is spread. The program emphasizes that the children are in control of their own health. In this program, children are taught that (1) while AIDS is a very serious disease, casual contact with children at home or school will not give them AIDS; (2) good health is something to be treasured, not taken for granted, and eating well, exercising, and not taking drugs affect their own good health; and (3) people with AIDS need help, compassion, and friendship. An information sheet accompanies this program.

Late Elementary/Middle School Although the lifestyles of most students at the late elementary/middle school level may not likely include risk behavior, a comprehensive AIDS education at this level would provide them knowledge and skill necessary to avoid risky behavior. Following are recommended audiovisuals for this grade level.

About AIDS. South Deerfield, MA: Channing L. Bete Co., Inc., 1987, 15 minutes. The program uses interviews with health authorities, individuals on the street concerning their beliefs about AIDS, and animated cartoons to describe the cause, prevention, and misinformation concerning AIDS. Additionally, this program provides the viewer with information about the tests that detect the presence of AIDS and the need for subsequent counseling for persons being tested. The program also identifies the types of behavior that can transmit the AIDS virus and offers suggestions for avoiding the possible consequences of that behavior. Two booklets, a leader's guide, and a poster accompanies this program.

AIDS: You Write the Prescription. Elizabethtown, PA: Continental Press, 1988, 27 minutes. This tape, which is intended for children in grades 3–6, features Dr. Dossett discussing AIDS and HIV infection with a group of elementary school students. The setting is a classroom with fourth and fifth grade students. Illustrations and cartoon characters are used to demonstrate points made by Dr. Dossett. The program defines AIDS and HIV infection, describes the stages of HIV infection that eventually result in AIDS, reviews the ways in which HIV infection is contracted, and discusses how to avoid getting infected with HIV. The accompanying 16-page user's guide outlines the videotape's contents, contains a glossary of terms, offers suggestions on how to use the videotape in class, and provides the names, addresses, and telephone numbers of sources of additional information.

Food for Thought. Washington Crossing, PA: Odyssey in Learning, 1988, 10 minutes. This program uses cartoon characters to present information about the AIDS virus. In this program, Drac, the grandson of Dracula, encounters a culture that contains the AIDS virus. Information is presented as Drac investigates what AIDS is. He learns that the virus is transmitted only by the exchange of body fluids, especially blood, and that such exchanges occur only by sharing IV drug equipment, from an infected mother to her infant, and by engaging in sexual intercourse. At the conclusion of the program Drac realizes that he should change his desire for blood because it could lead to AIDS infection. The tape also includes a 12-page AIDS Awareness Teacher's Curriculum Guide and six masters for handout sheets.

Understanding and Preventing AIDS. Chicago, IL: Children's Press, 1987, 13 minutes. This program has two parts. The first part identifies basic scientific information about the AIDS virus (what it is, different methods of transmission, prevention). Sexual abstinence among teenagers is also discussed. The second section discusses ways in which the sexually active youth can keep from contracting the virus. The accompanying information for the teacher includes student objectives, suggested readiness activities, follow-up activities, and toll-free hotlines and information sources. Throughout the program emphasis is placed on abstinence as the most effective way to avoid the AIDS virus.

Junior High/Senior High School Students who are at this stage of life appear to be the most endangered of all students for AIDS because of their risky lifestyles (e.g. drug use, unprotected sexual behavior, and prostitution). Most of the AIDS education must seek to help them to reduce their risk of infection with HIV by avoiding risky behavior, or peer pressure.

AIDS: An Enemy Among Us. Los Angeles, CA: Churchill Films, 1987, 45 minutes. This program provides information about the AIDS virus, how it is transmitted, methods of prevention, and diagnosis of infection with the AIDS virus. This made-for-television movie describes the life of a fictional teenager who receives a blood transfusion infected with the human immunodeficiency virus (HIV) during an operation. Attitudes of relatives, friends and school authorities are dramatized. The program discusses methods of prevention, including sexual abstinence, a mutually faithful relationship, avoiding sex with more than one person, and using condoms.

AIDS: Everything You Should Know. Van Nuys, CA: AIMS Media, 1988, 22 minutes. One of the problems faced by students at this level is denial. Most do not believe that they are susceptible to AIDS even if they engage in risky behaviors. This film provides the student a comprehensive education about the AIDS virus and how it is transmitted; it dispels the myths and unwarranted fear about the AIDS virus and how it is transmitted; it dispels the myths and unwarranted fear about the disease and suggests how students can protect themselves from the virus. This program, which is hosted by actress Whoopi Goldberg, is a mixture of discussions about AIDS by an ethnically diverse group of high school students, including presentations by health officials. Additionally, the program presents the facts that AIDS is not transmitted by casual contact in school or other public places, and is not conveyed through the air; nor is it spread by drinking fountains, toilet seats, doorknobs, hugging, sneezing, friendly kissing or coughing. Also, students are advised to be assertive when resisting peer pressure to engage in sex: "abstain from sexual contact until you can form a faithful monogamous relationship." A 12-page discussion guide is included.

AIDS: Wise, No Lies. New York, NY: New Day Films, 1988, 23 minutes. This program depends on individual testimonials to convey warning to teenagers about the results of behavior that can expose them to the AIDS virus. Ten individuals whose lives are affected by the AIDS virus express their thoughts, emotions, and experiences in dealing with the virus. The accompanying 35-page study guide is designed for a five-day lesson plan. It is preceded by basic facts on AIDS and followed by skill-building practice. The goals of the lesson plan are to establish a common foundation of basic facts regarding AIDS, to make AIDS and the implications of the disease real to young people and to identify and practice some of the skills relevant to AIDS prevention.

AIDS Risk? It's Your Choice! Ft. Worth, TX: American Institute for Teen AIDS Prevention, 1990, 35 minutes. This program depicts an education assembly on the human immunodeficiency virus (HIV) at the Polytechnic High School in Fort Worth, Texas. In this program, HIV and AIDS are discussed from a conceptual view, covering presentations on: (1) facts about HIV/AIDS, (2) students' personal risk, (3) avoiding infection, (4) inappropriate fears, and (5) how victims should be treated. This production is accompanied by a student brochure (*Don't Let AIDS Catch You: Straight Talk About AIDS*) and a teacher's brochure (*AIDS Education for Your Students*).

Choices: Learning About AIDS. Chicago, IL: National Safety Council, 1988, 20 minutes. This program is suitable for a racially and sexually mixed group of high school students and the various situations they find themselves in, particularly as they relate to the AIDS virus.

Don't Forget Sherrie. Washington, DC: American Red Cross, 1987, 32 minutes. This program, which is available through Modern Talking Picture Service, is available on loan from many local Red Cross chapters. The production investigates the emotions, concerns and lack of information high school students experience when confronted with the AIDS virus. This program features a largely black cast and dramatizes the effects of AIDS on black and urban youth. The storyline concentrates on a black male who discovers his former girlfriend, who used IV drugs, is dying of AIDS. This information causes him and his present girlfriend to consider whether they are at risk for the AIDS virus. There is a 22-page discussion guide that may be ordered separately.

In Control. Seattle, WA: Comprehensive Health Education Foundation, 1988, 27 minutes. This program is designed to help teenagers resist peer pressure to participate in behavior which may expose them to the AIDS virus. The tape is part of a multimedia instructional package on AIDS and HIV for high school students in grades 9–12. The program states that "it's not who you are but what you do with your body that places you at risk." Several "vignettes" are used to demonstrate common ways that teenagers are drawn into undesirable situations by friends and how to tactfully resist involvement in these situations.

A Letter from Brian. Washington, DC: American Red Cross, 1987, 27 minutes. This program depicts a female high school student who receives a letter from her former boyfriend that states he has AIDS. She and her present boyfriend must now confront their lack of knowledge about the disease. The program emphasizes the importance of not rushing into sexual intercourse. Those who engage in sex are encouraged to be monogamous and protect themselves by always using a condom. It also addresses teenagers' fears, needs, and misconceptions about AIDS. This program is available through Modern Talking Picture Service.

Ojos Que No Ven (Eyes That Fail to See). San Francisco, CA: Instituto Familiar de la Raza, 1987, 51 minutes. This tape will expose Hispanic students to AIDS information that is sensitive to their culture. The storyline of this production follows a woman whose co-worker is hospitalized with AIDS. Other characters include a homosexual male and a husband who spends the night with a prostitute. Even though the program deals with teenage sexuality, homosexuality and prostitution, it also discusses the closeted men in heterosexual marriages, and IV drug use. The program is "intended to represent more than an AIDS education tool; the producers hope that the Latino community will make AIDS part of its everyday consciousness and will be moved to care for and educate its people." A 32-page viewer guide accompanies this tape.

Straight Talk: David Talks to Teens About Drug Use and AIDS. New York, NY: New York Department of Health, 1989, 19 minutes. The program uses a question and answer format between an ex–IV drug user named David who has the AIDS virus and a group of teenagers to discuss AIDS. David explains what AIDS is and how it is transmitted, prevention measures, the relationship of AIDS to other sexually transmitted diseases, and what health behavior and types of sexual contact place a person at risk for getting the AIDS virus. David, who has AIDS, discusses his family's and friend's reactions to his having AIDS, how he started abusing drugs, how he felt when he learned he had the AIDS virus, his present emotional state and how drugs and AIDS have affected his life. In the process, teenagers are informed that there is no specific time, after infection, when the AIDS virus can be detected.

Taking Charge: You and AIDS. Berkeley, CA: Lodestar Productions, 1987, 16 minutes. This program deals with different ethnic groups (white, black, and Hispanic students) and is integrated with commentary by Dr. Marshall Kubota, and a discussion between students training to be AIDS peer educators with AIDS health educator Wendy Arnold. The program states that the AIDS virus is transmitted in semen, blood, and vaginal fluid, and that any sexually active person who engages in "risky" behavior is vulnerable to the AIDS virus. The AIDS virus is transmitted by sexual contact (vaginal and anal), the sharing of infected needles, perinatal processes, and contact with infected blood. Students reinforce that "it's cool to say no," and that it is wise to take relationships slowly. Prevention methods discussed include sexual abstinence, avoidance of

IV drug use and equipment, avoiding sex with multiple partners, and the use of condoms with spermicide.

Understanding AIDS: What Teens Need to Know. Pleasantville, NY: Sunburst Communications, 1988, 19 minutes. In this tape, a group of teenagers discuss AIDS while two physicians inject information. The physicians are Dr. Daren Hein, the Director of the Adolescent AIDS unit at Montefiore Medical Center in New York City, and Dr. Harvey Makadon, Director of Ambulatory Medical Services at Beth Israel Hospital in Boston. The doctors emphasize that AIDS is hard to catch and that the HIV virus is transmitted only by sexual intercourse (vaginal and anal), the sharing of IV drug equipment, perinatal processes, and HIV-infected blood transfusions. They also emphasize that the only sure ways of avoiding the AIDS virus are to abstain from sexual intercourse and to avoid the use of IV drugs.

Teacher Preparation The preparation of teachers is essential to the dissemination of appropriate information about AIDS. Teachers are also positioned to develop AIDS education curricula for their students. Consequently, they too must educate themselves about AIDS, HIV, and sexually transmitted diseases. The following audiovisuals will help prepare teachers to educate their students about AIDS.

AIDS: No Longer a Medical Mystery. Philadelphia, PA: Philadelphia School District, 1987, 29 minutes. This program provides information about the epidemiology, transmission, and prevention of the AIDS virus. The discussion includes the policies of the Philadelphia school system as they relate to students with AIDS. Basically, the school policy regarding HIV-infected students and employees states that infected persons are not automatically admitted or excluded from school but that a review of each case is necessary. Additional topics of discussion are high-risk groups for AIDS, the proper handling of blood spills in the school environment, and the use of school bathrooms and water fountains by AIDS-infected students.

AIDS: On the Front Line. Houston, TX: Houston Academy of Medicine, 1987, 23 minutes. The object of this program is to prepare teachers to instruct their students about AIDS. Information is presented on what AIDS is and its epidemiology in the United States and other countries. This program also emphasizes that adolescents are less knowledgeable than adults, are strongly influenced by their peers, are frequently involved with drugs or sexually active, and are less likely to modify their behavior. Also, teachers are encouraged to take parents' and community views into consideration when instructing students about their behavior. Teachers are urged to consider their own prejudices and feelings before presenting AIDS-related information.

AIDS: Suddenly Sex Has Become Very Dangerous. Cuero, TX: Goodday Video Productions, Inc., 1988, 30 minutes. The tape is a parents' and teachers' version that contains the entire "young people's" version, so that the adults can preview what the youngsters will be seeing. The program does not contain any graphic information about sex. Nor does it depict any methods of birth control besides sexual abstinence. This production is narrated by Annalee Jeffries, who explains that the tape that the youngsters will see is designed to modify their behavior and that the behavior modification cannot be completed without the help of the parents and teachers.

AIDS: What Every Teacher Must Know. Weston, CT: Instructional Media Institute, 1988, 76 minutes. This program is designed to develop skills, strategies, and information for teaching AIDS prevention. It is intended for teacher training and parent viewing; discretion is advised for children under 15 years of age. The video presents Veronica Skerker, a health consultant with the Connecticut State Department of Education, as she instructs a class of teachers and answers questions. The program is also intended to desensitize the subject of negative feeling toward AIDS carriers through effective training in handling AIDS information. These are presented in two segments: Part one presents factual information about AIDS and AIDS prevention. Part two offers recommendations for listening to, restating, and clarifying students' difficult questions about AIDS; for overcoming communication barriers; and for providing responses tailored to school policy and the students' grade level. Teachers are told that students should be encouraged to avoid alcohol and drugs, which weaken the immune system, and especially to avoid IV drug use. Several role-playing sessions are presented in which the instructor portrays students asking sensitive questions about AIDS and the teachers are to practice the skills presented in the video.

Universal Precautions Program. Roswell, GA: AMS Distributors, Inc., 1990, 11 minutes. This Universal Precautions Program (UPP) consists of two presentations subtitled (1) Origin and Purpose and (2) Precautions and Procedures. The first program describes the infectious viruses human immunodeficiency virus (HIV), Hepatitis B, and Cytomegalovirus as well as means of infection and modes of transmission. The program states that the common element between these diseases is that they are blood borne and spread through contact with body fluids. The second section of this presentation "discusses the chain of transmission: Infectious Agent, Exposure to Body Fluids, and Entering the Blood Stream and the means by which a person can break the chain and avoid exposure and contamination to these infectious diseases at the workplace." Specific behaviors that can promote self protection are mentioned. They include the use of disposable gloves, hand washing techniques, clean-up and disinfecting methods and proper disposal techniques.

We Owe It to Ourselves and to Our Children. Oakland, CA: National Native American AIDS Prevention Center, n.d., 8 minutes. This program was produced by the San Francisco–based Human Health Organization. It is designed for Native American communities. The film provides information on how AIDS is transmitted. This is an excellent film for teacher training because it is culturally sensitive.

Audiovisual Ordering Information

To order AIDS education audiovisuals, write or call the distributors listed below. In some cases, it may be possible to obtain preview copies.

Accent Presentations
990 Highland Drive
Suite 201
P.O. Box 1303
Solana Beach, CA 92075
(619) 755-1158

ACTA Publications
4848 North Clark Street
Chicago, IL 60640
(312) 271-1030

AIDS Education Project
Houston Academy of Medicine
113 M.D. Anderson Blvd.
Suite 400
Houston, TX 77030
(713) 790-1838

AIDS Films
50 West 34th Street
Suite 6B6
New York, NY 10001
(212) 629-6288

AIMS Media
6901 Woodley Avenue
Van Nuys, CA 91406-4878
(800) 367-2467

Alfred Higgins Productions, Inc.
9100 Sunset Blvd.
Los Angeles, CA 90069
(818) 762-3300

American Institute for Teen AIDS Prevention
P.O. Box 136116
Ft. Worth, TX 76136
(817) 237-0230

AMS Distributors, Inc.
P.O. Box 457
Rosewell, GA 30077

Barr Films
12801 Schabarum
P.O. Box 7878
Irwindale, CA 91706-7878
(818) 338-7878

Cannata Communications Corporation
7031 Grand Blvd.
Houston, TX 77054
(713) 748-1684

Channing L. Bete Co., Inc.
200 State Road
South Deerfield, MA 01373
(800) 628-7733

Children's Press
544 North Cumberland Avenue
Chicago, IL 60656
(312) 693-0800

Churchill Films
662 N. Robertson Blvd.
Los Angeles, CA 90069
(800) 334-7830

Comprehensive Health Education Foundation
22323 Pacific Highway South
Seattle, WA 98198-7253
(206) 824-2907

Continental Press
520 East Bainbridge
Elizabethtown, PA 17022
(800) 233-0759; (800) 847-0656

Coronet/MTI Film and Video
108 Wilmot Road
Deerfield, IL 60015
(800) 621-2131

Creative Media Group, Inc.
226 East High Street
Charlottesville, VA 22901
(804) 296-6138

Durrin Productions
1748 Kalorama Road, NW
Washington, DC 20009
(202) 387-6700

Goodday Video Productions, Inc.
P.O. Box 111
Cuero, TX 77954
(800) 221-1426; (512) 275-9141

Guidance Associates, Inc.
Communications Park
Box 3000
Mount Kisco, NY 10549-0900
(800) 431-1242; (914) 666-4100

Health Edco, Inc.
P.O. Box 21207
Waco, TX 76702
(800) 433-2677

Human Relations Media
175 Thomplins Avenue
Pleasantville, NY 10570
(800) 431-2050

Instituto Familiar de la Raza, Inc.
2515-24th Street, No. 2
San Francisco, CA 94110
(415) 647-4141

Instructional Media Institute
389 Newton Turnpike
Weston, CT 06883
(800) 243-5020

Light Video Television, Inc.
21 Highland Circle
Needham, MA 02194

Lodestar Productions
P.O. Box 8226
Berkeley, CA 94707
(415) 525-7516

Michelle, Ogilvy and Mather Public Affairs
1901 L Street, NW
Suite 320
Washington, DC 20036
(202) 466-7590

Milestone Productions
1565 16th Avenue
San Francisco, CA 91422

Modern Talking Picture Service
5000 Park Street North
St. Petersburg, FL 33709
(800) 237-4599; (813) 541-5763

National Native American AIDS Prevention Center
3515 Grand Avenue
Suite 100
Oakland, CA 94610
(510) 444-2051

National Safety Council (NSC)
444 North Michigan Avenue
Chicago, IL 60611
(800) 621-7619; (312) 527-4800

New Day Films
853 Broadway
Suite 1210
New York, NY 10003
(212) 477-4604

New Dimension Media
85895 Lorane Highway
Eugene, OR 97405
(800) 288-4456

New York Department of Health
Division of Health Promotion
Corning Tower
Room 1084
Empire State Plaza
Albany, NY 12237

Odyssey in Learning
3 Bankers Drive
Washington Crossing, PA 18977
(215) 493-1675

Peer Education Health Resources
P.O. Box 3262
Minneapolis, MN 55403
(612) 823-6257

Perennial Education, Inc.
930 Pitner Avenue
Evanston, IL 60202
(800) 323-9084

Philadelphia School District
AIDS Education
Room 402
Stevens Administrative Center
Spring Garden Street at 13th Street
Philadelphia, PA 19123
(215) 351-7131

Printed Matter, Inc.
P.O. Box 15246, NE
Atlanta, GA 30333
(404) 377-3927

Pyramid Film and Video
2801 Colorado Avenue
Santa Monica, CA 90404
(800) 421-2304; (213) 828-7577

ReBab Studio
99 Orchid S.W.
Rio Rancho, NM 87124
(505) 891-8410

San Francisco AIDS Foundation
333 Valencia Street
4th Floor
San Francisco, CA 94103

Select Media, Inc.
74 Varick Street
Suite 305
New York, NY 10013
(212) 431-8923

STOP AIDS
1640 North Gower Street
Hollywood, CA 90028

Sunburst Communications
Room KH20
101 Castleton Street
Pleasantville, NY 10570-3498
(800) 431-1934

WETA-TV
Educational Activities Office
P.O. Box 2626
Washington, DC 20013
(800) 445-1964

References

Campeau, P. L. (1974). "Selective Review of the Results of Research on the Use of Audio-visual Media to Teach Adults." *Audio-Visual Communications Review,* 22:5–40.

Center for Population Options (1989, April). "The Changing Face of AIDS: Adolescents and HIV Infection (Editorial Memorandum)." Washington, DC: CPO.

____ (1988, November). "HIV and AIDS: How Can I Protect Myself? A Unit of HIV Infection for the Life Planning Curriculum." Washington, DC: CPO.

Centers for Disease Control (1988, January 28). "Guidelines for Effective School Health Education to Prevent the Spread of AIDS." *MMWR;* 37 (supp. no. S-2).

Kreps, G. (1988). "Relational Communication in Health Care." *Southern Speech Communication Journal,* 43:344–359.

Nugent, G. C. (1982). "Pictures, Audio, and Print: Symbolic Representation and Effect on Learning." *Educational Communication and Technology,* 30:163–74.

Rowher, W. D., and Matz, R. (1975). "Improving Aural Comprehension in White and Black Children: Pictures-vs-Print." *Journal of Experimental Child Psychology,* 19: 23–26.

Sawyer, R. G., and Beck, K. H. (1991, March-April). "Effects of Videotapes on Perceived Susceptibility to HIV/AIDS Among University Freshmen." *Health Values,* 15(2):31–40.

Vasu, E. S., and Howe, A. C. (1989). "The Effect of Visual and Verbal Modes of Presentation on Children's Retention of Images and Words." *Journal of Research in Science Teaching,* 26:401–407.

Chapter Fifteen

Resources Directory for HIV/AIDS Information, Education and Prevention

A. ODASUO ALALI

Following is a selected resources directory that public schools can use to build partnerships with government and nongovernmental organizations, as well as educational and research institutions that provide HIV/AIDS information, and education and prevention services. The selection of these organizations was based on the author's perception of their commitment to the prevention of AIDS through public awareness and improved understanding of the disease.

This directory is divided into nine resource categories: national organizations, state public health departments, national school health programs, state school health programs, local school health programs, regional AIDS education and training centers, philanthropic organizations, expert review panels, and brochure screening consultants.

Each organization or institution provides a variety of services that include public awareness programs, educational materials to assist teachers, advocacy for AIDS funding, support services, informational clearinghouses and hotlines, training programs, brochure screening, pamphlets, and other relevant educational publications and instructional materials. Public schools can augment their HIV/AIDS education programs through collaborative ventures with these organizations.

The philanthropic organizations provide financial support for school-based programs that emphasize education and prevention of AIDS. This directory identifies each organization by name, address, telephone number, and, when possible, fax number. They are subject to change.

1. National

AIDS Action Council
1875 Connecticut Avenue
Suite 700
Washington, DC 20009
(202) 986-1300; Fax: (202) 986-1345

AIDS Coalition to Unleash Power (ACT UP)
135 W. 29th Street, 10th Fl.
New York, NY 10001
(212) 564-2437

AIDS Education Project
Institute for Development Training
P.O. Box 2522
Chapel Hill, NC 27515-2522
(919) 967-0563

The Alan Guttmacher Institute
2010 Massachusetts Avenue, NW
Washington, DC 20036
(202) 296-4021

American Enterprise Institute for Public Policy Research (AEI)
1150 17th St. NW
Washington, DC 20036
(202) 862-5800

American Foundation for AIDS Research (AmFAR)
40 West 57th St.
New York, NY 10019
(212) 333-3118

American Institute for Teens AIDS Prevention
P.O. Box 136116
Fort Worth, TX 76136

American Red Cross National Headquarters
AIDS Education Office
1730 D St., NW
Washington, DC 20006
(202) 737-8300

Center for Population Options (CPO)
National Office
1025 Vermont Avenue, NW
Suite 210
Washington, DC 20005
(202) 347-5700; Fax (202) 347-2263

Centers for Disease Control
AIDS Information Office
Atlanta, GA 30333
(404) 329-2891

The Citizen Commission on AIDS
121 Avenue of the Americas
6th Floor
New York, NY 10013
(212) 925-5290

COSSMHO
Coalition of Hispanic Health and Human Services Organizations
1030 15th St. NW
Washington, DC 20005
(202) 371-2100; (800) AIDS-123 (hotline)

George Washington University
Intergovernmental Health Policy Project
20111 St., NW
Suite 200
Washington, DC 20006
(202) 872-1445

The Kids on the Block, Inc.
9385-C Germig Lane
Columbia, MD 21046
(800) 368-KIDS

Lambda Legal Defense & Education Fund
666 Broadway
New York, NY 10012
(212) 995-8585

National AIDS Hotline
(800) 342-AIDS
(7 days a week, 24 hours a day)

National AIDS Hotline Classroom
[for brochure about services, call (800) 342-AIDS]

National AIDS Information Clearinghouse (NAIC)
P.O. Box 6003
Rockville, MD 20850
(800) 342-AIDS; (800) 458-5231

National AIDS Network (NAN)
1012 14th St. NW
Suite 601
Washington, DC 20005
(202) 347-0390

National Association of People with AIDS (NAPWA)
2025 I St. NW
Suite 415
Washington, DC 20006
(202) 347-1317

National Gay and Lesbian Task Force
1517 U St., NW
Washington, DC 20009
(202) 332-6483

National Hemophilia Foundation
SoHo Bldg.
110 Greene St., Rm. 406
New York, NY 10012
(212) 219-8180

National Leadership Coalition on AIDS
1150 17th St.
Suite 202
Washington, DC 20036
(202) 429-0930

National Minority AIDS Council
714 G St., SE
P.O. Box 28574 (20038)
Washington, DC 20003
(202) 544-1076

National Native American AIDS Prevention Center
Center for Women Policy Studies
5266 Boyd Avenue
Oakland, CA 94618
(415) 654-2093

Peer Education Health Resources
P.O. Box 3262
Minneapolis, MN 55403
(612) 823-6257

Planned Parenthood Federation of America, Inc.
810 7th Avenue
New York, NY 10019
(212) 261-4633; Fax (212) 245-1845

Project Inform (PI)
347 Dolores St., Suite 301
San Francisco, CA 94110
(800) 822-7422
San Francisco AIDS Foundation
P.O. Box 6182
San Francisco, CA 94101-6182
(415) 861-3397

Sex Information and Education Council of the U.S. (SIECUS)
130 West 42nd Street, Suite 2500
New York, NY 10036
(212) 819-9770; Fax (212) 819-9776

U.S. Conference of Mayors
AIDS Program
1620 Eye St., NW
4th Floor
Washington, DC 20006
(202) 293-7330

Women's AIDS Project (WAP)
8235 Santa Monica Blvd., Suite 201
West Hollywood, CA 90046
(213) 650-1508

2. State Public Health Departments (alphabetical by state)

Alabama Dept. of Health
AIDS Program
State Office Building, Room 662
434 Monroe St.
Montgomery, AL 36130
(205) 261-5017; (800) 228-0469

Alaska Dept. of Health
AIDS Health Program
3601 C St.
Anchorage, AK 99524
(907) 561-4406

Arizona Dept. of Health
Office of Health Education
431 North 24th St.
Phoenix, AZ 85008
(602) 230-5836; (800) 344-1540

Arkansas Dept. of Health
AIDS Activities
4815 West Markham
Little Rock, AR 72205
(501) 661-2135; (800) 445-7720

California Dept. of Health
Office of AIDS
P.O. Box 160146
Sacramento, CA 95816
(916) 445-0553; (800) 367-2437 (Northern Cal)

Colorado Dept. of Health
AIDS Education Risk Reduction Program
4210 East 11th St.
Denver, CO 80220
(303) 331-8320

Connecticut Dept. of Health
AIDS Program
150 Washington St.
Hartford, CT 06112
(203) 566-5058; (203) 566-1157

D.C. Commission of Public Health
Division of AIDS Education
1875 Connecticut Ave., NW
Room 838-C
Washington, DC 20009
(202) 673-3425; (202) 332-AIDS

Delaware Dept. of Health and Social Services
AIDS Program Office
3000 Newport Gap Pike
Building G
Wilmington, DE 19808
(302) 995-8422

Florida Dept. of Health-Rehabilitation
Health Education and Risk Reduction
1317 Winewood Blvd.
Building 6, Room 453
Tallahassee, FL 32399
(904) 487-2478; (800) FLA-AIDS

Georgia Dept. of Human Resources
STD Control Program
878 Peachtree St., NE
Atlanta, GA 30309
(404) 894-5147; (800) 551-2728

Hawaii Dept. of Health Public
Public Health Education
3627 Kilauea Ave.
Honolulu, HI 96816
(808) 735-5303; (808) 922-1313

Idaho Dept. of Health and Welfare
AIDS Program
450 West State St.
Boise, ID 83720
(208) 334-5930

Illinois Dept. of Health
Health Education
525 West Jefferson
Springfield, IL 62761
(217) 782-2016; (800) 243-2438

Indiana Dept. of Public Health
Office of AIDS Activity
1330 West Michigan
Indianapolis, IN 46206
(317) 633-8406

Iowa Dept. of Public Health
AIDS Education
Lucas Building
3rd Floor
Des Moines, IA 50319
(515) 281-4938; (800) 532-3301

Kansas Dept. of Health and Environment
Office of Health Education
Forbes Field Building 321
Room 13
Topeka, KS 66620
(913) 296-5587; (800) 232-0040

Kentucky Dept. for Health Services
AIDS Health Education
275 E. Main St.
Frankfort, KY 40621
(502) 564-4804; (800) 654-AIDS

Louisiana Office of Prevention Medicine and Public Health Services
325 Loyola Ave.
Room 615
New Orleans, LA 70012
(504) 568-5005; (800) 999-4379

Maine Bureau of Health
Office on AIDS
Station House, Station 11
Augusta, ME 04333
(207) 289-3591; (800) 851-AIDS

Maryland Dept. of Health and Mental Hygiene Epidemiology
201 West Preston St.
Baltimore, MD 21201
(301) 225-6707; (800) 638-6252

Massachusetts Dept. of Public Health
AIDS Health Education
150 Tremont St.
Boston, MA 02111
(617) 727-0368; (800) 235-2331

Michigan Dept. of Health
Special Office of AIDS Prevention
3423 N. Logan
Lansing, MI 48909
(517) 335-8371; (800) 872-AIDS

Minnesota Dept. of Health
AIDS Program
717 S.E. Delaware St.
Minneapolis, MN 55440
(612) 623-5414; (800) 248-AIDS

Mississippi Dept. of Health
AIDS Education Program
P.O. Box 1700
Jackson, MS 39215
(601) 960-7725; (800) 826-2961

Missouri Dept. of Health
AIDS Program
P.O. Box 570
Jefferson City, MO 65102
(314) 751-6438

Montana Dept. of Health and Environmental Services
AIDS Program
Cogswell Building
Helena, MT 59260
(406) 444-2457

Nebraska Dept. of Health
AIDS Prevention Program
P.O. Box 95007
Lincoln, NE 68509
(402) 471-2937; (800) 782-2437

Nevada State Health Division
Dept. of Human Resources
505 East King St., Room 200
Carson City, NV 89710
(702) 885-4800

New Hampshire Dept. of Health and Welfare
6 Hazen Dr.
Concord, NH 03301
(603) 271-4490

New Jersey Dept. of Health
AIDS Division
C.N. 360, 363 West State St.
Trenton, NJ 08625
(609) 984-6000; (800) 624-2377

New Mexico Dept. of Health and Environment Epidemiology
P.O. Box 968
Santa Fe, NM 87504
(505) 827-0086

New York State Dept. of Health
AIDS Institute
1315 Empire State Plaza, 25th Floor, Room 2580
Albany, NY 12237
(518) 474-8160

North Carolina Health Dept.
AIDS Control Program
P.O. Box 2091
Raleigh, NC 27602
(919) 733-3419

North Dakota Dept. of Health
AIDS Project
State Capitol Building
Bismark, ND 58505
(701) 224-8378; (800) 592-1861

Ohio Dept. of Health
AIDS Activity Unit
246 North High St.
Columbus, OH 43266
(614) 466-5480; (800) 332-AIDS

Oklahoma Dept. of Health
STD Division
P.O. Box 53551
Oklahoma City, OK 73152
(405) 271-5601

Oregon Dept. of Health
AIDS Program
1400 Southwest 5th St.
Room 710
Portland, OR 97201
(503) 229-5792

Pennsylvania Dept. of Health
Disease Control
P.O. Box 90
Harrisburg, PA 17108
(717) 787-3350; (800) 692-7254

Puerto Rico Dept. of Health
Call Box STD, Caparra Heights Station
San Juan, PR 00922
(809) 754-8118

Rhode Island Dept. of Health
AIDS Control Program
75 Davis
Room 105
Providence, RI 02908
(401) 277-2362; (401) 277-6502

South Carolina Dept. of Health
AIDS Project
2600 Bull St.
Columbia, SC 29201
(803) 734-5482; (800) 322-AIDS

South Dakota Dept. of Health
AIDS Program
523 East Capital
Pierre, SD 57501
(605) 773-3357; (800) 472-2180

Tennessee Dept. of Health and Environment—Disease Control
100 9th Ave. North
Nashville, TN 37219
(615) 741-7387; (800) 342-AIDS

Texas Dept. of Health
Epidemiology–Health Promotion
100 West 49th St.
Austin, TX 78756
(512) 458-7405

Utah Dept. of Health
Epidemiology
288 North, 1460 West
P.O. Box 16660
Salt Lake City, UT 84116
(801) 538-6191; (801) 466-9976; (800) 843-9388

Vermont Dept. of Health
AIDS Education
60 Main St.
P.O. Box 70
Burlington, VT 05402
(802) 863-7245; (800) 882-AIDS

Virgin Islands Dept. of Health
AIDS Committee
P.O. Box 7309
St. Thomas, VI 00801
(809) 776-8311

Virginia Dept. of Health
AIDS Activity Program
109 Governor St.
Room 722
Richmond, VA 23219
(804) 786-6267; (800) 533-4148

Washington Dept. of Health
Epidemiology–AIDS Program
1610 Northeast 150th St.
Seattle, WA 98155
(206) 361-2888

West Virginia Dept. of Health
151 11th Ave.
South Charleston, WV 25303
(304) 348-5358; (800) 624-8244

Wisconsin Dept. of Health and Social Services
AIDS Program
1 West Wilson St.
P.O. Box 309
Madison, WI 53701
(608) 267-5287; (800) 334-AIDS

Wyoming Division of Health and Medical Services

AIDS Program
Hathaway Building
4th Floor
Cheyenne, WY 82002
(307) 777-7953

3. National School Health Programs (alphabetical by title)

AIDS Education for Incarcerated Youth
Harrison, E.A.
National Commission on Correctional Health Care
2000 North Racine
Suite 3500
Chicago, IL 60614
(312) 528-0818

AIDS Education Out-of-School Youth
Bogan, W. A.
National Coalition of Hispanic and Human Services Organizations (COSSMHO)
Division of National Programs
1030 15th Street, NW
Suite 1053
Washington, DC 20005
(202) 371-2100

AIDS Education Program for Colleges and Universities
Downey, P. A.
American College Health Association
15879 Crabbs Branch Way
Rockville, MD 20855
(301) 762-6102

AIDS Education Training Project for Colleges of Teacher Education
Cooney, J. L.
American College Health Association
15879 Crabbs Branch Way
Rockville, MD 20855
(301) 762-6102

American Association of School Administrators AIDS Education Initiative
Jones, E. H.; Ingraham, G. C.
American Association of School Administrators
1801 North Moore Street
Arlington, VA 22209
(703) 875-0728; (703) 875-0719

American Federation of Teachers AIDS Education Project
Nayman, L.
American Federation of Teachers
Department of Organization
555 New Jersey Avenue, NW
Washington, DC 20001
(202) 879-4548

American Medical Association Youth HIV Education Project
Fleming, M.
American Medical Association
535 North Dearborn Street
Chicago, IL 60610
(312) 645-5315

Council of Chief State School Officers HIV/Comprehensive School Health Program
Brown, C. G.
Council of Chief State School Officers
Resource Center on Educational Equity
400 North Capitol Street, NW
Suite 379
Washington, DC 20001
(201) 393-8159

HIV Education: Interdisciplinary, Multicultural Approaches for Students and Teachers
Smith, B.; Musillo, C.
American Alliance for Health, Physical Education, Recreation and Dance
Association for the Advancement of Health Education
1900 Association Drive
Reston, VA 22091
(703) 476-3441

Increasing the Number of Schools Providing HIV Education to Rural School-Age Populations
National Rural and Small Schools Consortium
National Rural Development Institute
Western Washington University—MH 359

Bellingham, WA 98225
(206) 676-3576

Local Schools Boards and HIV Education
Proposal to Provide Training and Resources to Local School Board Members to Promote HIV Education in the Nation's Public Schools
Gaddy, D.
National School Boards Association
1680 Duke Street
Alexandria, VA 22314
(703) 838-6722

National Campaign to Increase the Number of States Providing Comprehensive Leadership to Promote Effective HIV Education
Sullivan, C.
National Association of State Boards of Education
1012 Cameron Street
Alexandria, VA 22314
(703) 684-4000

National Coalition of Advocates for Students HIV/AIDS Education Project
National Coalition of Advocates for Students
100 Boylston Street
Suite 737
Boston, MA 12116
(617) 357-8507

National Education Association HIV Education and Training Project
Williams, J. H.
National Education Association
Health Information Network
100 Colony Square
Suite 200
Atlanta, GA 30361

National Organization of Black County Officials AIDS Education Project
Jones, C.
National Organization of Black County Officials
440 First Street, NW
Suite 500
Washington, DC 20001
(202) 347-6953

National PTA AIDS Education Project
Woerner, R.
National PTA
700 North Rush Street
Chicago, IL 60611
(312) 787-0977

Safe Choices Projects: HIV/AIDS Prevention /Education to School Aged Youth People Who Do Not Attend School
Bucy, J. P.
National Network of Runaway and Youth Services, Inc.
1400 I Street, NW
Suite 330
Washington, DC 20005
(202) 682-4114

School-Based HIV Education: A Multidisciplinary Approach to Prevention
David, D.; Kerr, D.
American School Health Association
7263 State Route 43
P.O. Box 708
Kent, OH 44240
(216) 678-1601

Teaching AIDS Training Project
Ludlow, S. O.
ETR Associates
Training Department
4 Carbonero Way
Scotts Valley, CA 95066
(408) 438-4060

Working with National Youth-Serving, Youth-Employment and Education Organizations to Develop and Expand Adolescent HIV Prevention Programs
Wigfall-Williams, W.
Center for Population Options
1025 Vermont Avenue, NW
Suite 210
Washington, DC 20005
(202) 347-5700; Fax: (202) 347-2263

4. State School Health Programs (alphabetical by state)

Alabama State Department of Education Plan of Action or HIV/AIDS Education
Barton, M.
Alabama State Department of Education
Student Instructional Services Division
481 State Office Building
Montgomery, AL 36130
(205) 261-5240

State Education Agency Programs for School Health Education to Prevent the Spread of HIV
Mehrkens, H.
Alaska State Department of Education
Office of Basic Education
P.O. Box F
Juneau, AK 99811-0500
(907) 465-2841

American Samoa AIDS/HIV Prevention and Education Program
Aab, R.
American Samoa Government Department of Education
P.O. Box DOE
Pago, Pago, American Samoa 96779
(684) 633-5237

School Health Education AIDS/HIV Prevention
Henderson, B.
Arizona State Department of Education
Comprehensive Health Unit
1535 W. Jefferson
Phoenix, AZ 85007
(602) 524-4273

State and Local Programs for School Health Education to Prevent the Spread of HIV in Arkansas
Towery, M.
Arkansas State Department of Education
Curriculum and Assessment Section
4 Capitol Mall
Little Rock, AR 72201
(501) 682-3537

AIDS Education in California Schools
Ryan, R.
California State Department of Education
Critical Health Initiatives
721 Capitol Mall
Sacramento, CA 95814
(916) 322-4018

The Colorado Program for School Health Education to Prevent the Spread of HIV
Sandau-Christopher, D.
Colorado State Department of Education
Office of Federal Relations
201 East Colfax Avenue
Denver, CO 80203
(303) 866-6664

AIDS Prevention Project
Brainerd, E.
Connecticut State Department of Education
Division of Education Support Services
P.O. Box 2219
Hartford, CT 06145
(203) 638-4228

Delaware State Program for School Health Education on HIV
Vincent, E. P.; Arns, J.
Delaware State Department of Public Instruction
Instructional Services
P.O. Box 1402
Townsend Building
Dover, DE 19903
(302) 736-4886

School Health Education to Prevent the Spread of AIDS
Freeman, V. L.; Sadler, J.
District of Columbia Public Schools
Lovejoy School
400 12th Street, NE
Washington, DC 20002
(202) 724-4930; (202) 724-4008

State and Local Programs for School Health Education to Prevent the Spread of AIDS
Routh, D.; Waters, M.

Florida State Department of Education
Office of Policy Research and Improvement
Knott Building
Tallahassee, FL 32399
(904) 488-1611; (904) 488-7835

HIV Grant Program
Stalvey, J. R.
Georgia State Board of Education
Division of General Instruction
1952 Twin Towers East
Atlanta, GA 30334-5040
(404) 656-2414

School Health Education to Prevent the Spread of HIV/AIDS Among Our Islandwide Students Grades K–12 in the Public and Private Schools
Basa, D. M.

Guam Department of Education
Division of Curriculum and Instruction
P.O. Box DE
Agana, Guam 96910
(671) 472-8901, Ext. 500

AIDS Education in Hawaii
Horluchi, A.
Hawaii State Department of Education
Office of Instructional Services
P.O. Box 2360
Honolulu, HI 96804
(808) 395-8810

Idaho AIDS Education Program
Hummer, J.
Idaho State Department of Education
Bureau of Instruction
650 W. State Street
Boise, ID 83720
(208) 334-2281

School Health Education to Prevent the Spread of HIV
Sampson, J. R.
Illinois State Board of Education
School Improvement/Curriculum Improvement
100 North First Street
Springfield, IL 62777
(217) 782-2826

Indiana AIDS Education Program
Usher, P. L.
Indiana State Department of Education
Student Services, Room 229
State House
Indianapolis, IN 46204-2798
(317) 232-9100

Iowa AIDS Education Program
Edge, E.
Iowa State Department of Education
Bureau of Instruction and Curriculum
Grimes State Office Building
Des Moines, IA 50319-0146
(515) 242-6023

Kansas Program for School Health Education to Prevent the Spread of AIDS and Sexually Transmitted Diseases
Moore, R.
Kansas State Department of Education
120 E. 10th Street
Topeka, KS 66612-1103
(913) 296-3851

Kentucky AIDS Prevention Education
Mudd, I.
Kentucky State Department of Education
Division of Curriculum and Staff Development
Capital Plaza Tower
18th Floor
Frankfort, KY 40601
(502) 564-2106

State Program for Health Education to Prevent the Spread of AIDS
Frost, D. O.
Louisiana State Department of Education
626 North Fourth Street
Room 704
Baton Rouge, LA 70804
(504) 342-5431

State AIDS Education Program
Richards, W. H.
Maine State Department of Educational and Cultural Services
Bureau of Instruction
State House Station #23
Augusta, ME 04333

School Health Education to Prevent the Spread of AIDS
Henke, R.
Maryland State Department of Education
Division of Instruction
200 W. Baltimore Street
Baltimore, MD 21201
(301) 333-2318

Massachusetts AIDS Program
Haug-Simons, C.
Massachusetts State Department of Education
Division of School Programs
Bureau of Student Development and Health
1385 Hancock Street
Quincy, MA 02169
(617) 770-7593

State Program for School Health Education to Prevent the Spread of HIV
Jubb, W.
Michigan State Department of Education
Comprehensive School Health Unit
School Program Services
P.O. Box 30008
Lansing, MI 48909
(517) 373-2589

State Education Agency Programs to Prevent the Spread of HIV
DuVander, S.
Minnesota State Department of Education
AIDS Prevention and Risk Reduction
519 Capitol Square Building
550 Cedar Street
St. Paul, MN 55101
(612) 296-1431

HIV Education and Prevention
Bariow, J.
Mississippi State Department of Education
Bureau of Instructional Services
P.O. Box 771
Jackson, MS 39205-0771
(601) 359-3778

School Health Education to Prevent the Spread of AIDS Project
Baker, O.
Missouri State Department of Elementary and Secondary Education
Health Education Section
P.O. Box 480
Jefferson City, MO 65102
(314) 751-4234

Montana AIDS Education Program
Sartorius, S.
Montana State Office Public Instruction
Curriculum Services Unit
Capitol Building
Helena, MT 59620
(406) 444-4434

State and Local Education Agency-Programs for School Health Education to Prevent the Spread of AIDS
Owens-Nauslar, J.
Nebraska State Department of Education
Curriculum Services
301 Centennial Mall South
P.O. Box 94987
Lincoln, NE 68509
(402) 471-4334

HIV Public Education State Plan
Bacon, R. J.
Nevada State Department of Education
400 W. King Street
Capitol Complex
Carson City, NV 89710
(702) 885-3136

Program to Prevent the Spread of HIV Infection Among School-Aged Youth
Holt, K.; Ewert, W.
New Hampshire State Department of Education
Division of Instructional Services
101 Pleasant Street
Concord, NH 03301
(603) 271-2632

Cooperative Agreement for AIDS Prevention Education
Lindaman, A.
New Jersey State Department of Education
Division of General Academic Education

225 West State Street, CN 500
Trenton, NJ 08625
(609) 984-1890

School Health Education to Prevent the Spread of Human Immunodeficiency Virus
Sheffield, A.
New York State Education Department
Bureau of School Health Education and Services
Room 964 EBA
Albany, NY 12234
(518) 474-1491

Programs for School Health Education to Prevent the Spread of AIDS
Frye, R.
North Carolina State Department of Public Instruction
Education Building
116 W. Edenton Street
Raleigh, NC 27603-1712
(919) 733-3906

AIDS School Health Education Project
DeRemer, C.
North Dakota State Department of Public Instruction
State Capitol
600 E. Boulevard Avenue
Bismarck, ND 58505
(701) 224-2514

School Health Education to Prevent the Spread of AIDS
Schiraldi, F. L.
Ohio State Department of Education
Curriculum and Instruction Section
Division of Elementary and Secondary Education
Room 1005
65 South Front Street
Columbus, OH 43266-0308
(614) 466-2211

AIDS/HIV Prevention Education
Potts, H.; Richter, J.
Oklahoma State Department of Education
AIDS/HIV Prevention Education
2500 North Lincoln Boulevard
Oklahoma City, OK 73105-4599
(405) 521-2808; (405) 521-3361

Oregon HIV/AIDS Prevention Education Program
Christensen, A. A.
Oregon State Department of Education
Grants Management Branch
700 Pringle Parkway, S.E.
Salem, OR 97310
(503) 378-3615

Stop AIDS Via Education (SAVE)
Sutter, M. D.
Pennsylvania State Department of Education
Bureau of Curriculum and Instruction
333 Market Street
Dauphin County
Harrisburg, PA 17126-0333
(717) 787-9862

Accurate Information Delivery Services (AIDS) Vs. AIDS Project
Morales, C. M.
Puerto Rico Department of Education
P.O. Box 759
Hato Rey, PR 00919
(809) 756-5820

AIDS Prevention Project for School-Aged Youth to Prevent the Spread of AIDS
Costa, E. T.
Rhode Island State Department of Education
School Support Services
22 Hayes Street
Providence, RI 02908
(401) 277-2638

State and Local Education Agency Programs for Health Education to Prevent the Spread of HIV
Hynds, W. B.; Slater, A.
South Carolina State Department of Education
Curriculum Development Section
General Education
1429 Senate Street
801 Rutledge Building
Columbia, SC 29201
(803) 734-8366

Project SPACE: Statewide Prevention of AIDS Through Collaborative Efforts
Carr, M.
South Dakota State Department of Education and Cultural Affairs
Division of Education
AIDS Education
700 Governors Drive
Pierre, SD 57501-2293
(605) 773-3261

HIV/AIDS Education
Word, E. R.
Tennessee State Department of Education
Curriculum and Instruction
Cordell Hull Building
Fourth Floor, North Wing
Nashville, TN 37219
(615) 741-7856

Texas AIDS Prevention Education Project
Thomas, S. M.
Texas State Education Agency
Comprehensive School Health Programs
1701 North Congress
Austin, TX 78701
(512) 463-9501

AIDS Education Implementation in Schools Grades 3–12
Peterson, M.
Utah State Office of Education
Operations Division
Curriculum Section
250 East 500 South
Salt Lake City, UT 84111
(801) 538-7864

State and Local Education Agency Programs for School Health Education to Prevent the Spread of AIDS
Simpson, S.
Vermont State Department of Education
Basic Education
120 State Street
Montpelier, VT 05602
(802) 828-3111

National Programs for School Health Education to Prevent the Spread of AIDS
Tye, S.
Virgin Islands Department of Education
4446 Kongens Gade
St. Thomas, VI 00802
(809) 774-0100, Ext. 233

School Health Education to Prevent the Spread of AIDS
Bentley, J. L.
Virginia State Department of Education
P.O. Box 6Q
Richmond, VA 23216-2060
(804) 225-2866

Washington State Program for Health Education to Prevent the Spread of AIDS
Baldwin, P.
Washington State Office of the Superintendent of Public Instruction
Special Services and Professional Programs
Old Capitol Building, MS/FG-11
Olympia, WA 98504
(206) 753-2744

AIDS/HIV Prevention Education for West Virginia
Zsdosky, L.; Parr, N.
West Virginia State Department of Education
Bureau of General, Special, and Professional Education
Capitol Complex, B-309
Charleston, WV 25305
(304) 348-8830

AIDS/HIV Prevention Education Within Wisconsin Schools
Erpenbach, W.
Wisconsin State Department of Public Instruction
Bureau for Pupil Services
P.O. Box 7841
125 South Webster Street
Madison, WI 53707-7841
(608) 266-8960

State/Local AIDS School Health Education
Stowers, L.

Wyoming State Department of Education
Certification, Accreditation and Program Services
2300 Capitol Avenue
Hathaway Building
Cheyenne, WY 82001
(307) 777-6808

5. Local School Health Programs (alphabetical by locality)

AIDS Prevention Education in Baltimore City Schools
Bowden, A.
Baltimore (Maryland) City Public Schools
Office of Science and Health Education
200 East North Avenue
Baltimore, MD 21202
(301) 396-8573

AIDS Education Program
Grady, M. I.
Boston (Massachusetts) Public Schools
Department of Instructional Services
Boston Public Schools
26 Court Street
Boston, MA 02108
(617) 726-6200, Ext. 5192

School Health Education Program to Prevent the Spread of HIV
Sweigart, B.; Scalise, D. S.
Broward County School Board (Ft. Lauderdale, FL)
Comprehensive Health Education Department
The School Board of Broward County, Florida
1320 S.W. 4th Street
Ft. Lauderdale, FL 33312
(305) 760-7477

Cooperative Agreement to Support School Health Education to Prevent the Spread of AIDS
Bryant, P.
Chicago (Illinois) Public Schools
Department of Government Funded Programs
Chicago Public Schools
P.O. Box 699005
Chicago, IL 60609
(312) 890-8147

Dade County Public Schools HIV Information and Education Program
McIntosh, P. B.
Dade County School Board (Miami, FL)
Office of Federal Projects Administration
The School Board of Dade County, FL
1450 N.E. 2nd Avenue
Miami, Dade County, FL 33132
(305) 376-1704

Program for School Health Education to Prevent the Spread of AIDS
Simpson, P. E.
Dallas (Texas) Independent School District
Curriculum and Instructional Support
Dallas Independent School District
3700 Ross Avenue
Dallas County
Dallas, TX 75204
(214) 824-1620

School Health Education to Prevent the Spread of AIDS
Schonhaut, S.
Denver (Colorado) Public Schools
School District #1
Office of Federal/External Resources
Denver Public Schools
School District #1
900 Grant Street
Denver, CO 80203
(303) 837-1000, Ext. 2546

School Health Education to Prevent the Spread of AIDS
St. Paul, E. A.
Jersey City (New Jersey) Board of Education
Department of Support Programs
Jersey City Board of Education
346 Claremont Avenue
Jersey City, NJ 07305
(201) 915-6135

AIDS Prevention Project
Rich, R.

Los Angeles (California) Unified School District
Los Angeles Unified School District
Office of Instruction (Health Education)
450 North Grand Avenue
Room A-319
Los Angeles, CA 90012
(213) 625-6411

Health Education to Prevent the Spread of AIDS
Abelson, G.
New York City (New York) Board of Education
New York City Board of Education
Health, Physical Education, and School Sports
110 Livingston Street
Brooklyn (Kings), NY 11201
(718) 935-4140

School Health Education Project to Prevent the Spread of AIDS
Savage, G. B.
Newark (New Jersey) Board of Education
Newark Board of Education
Division of Grants Development
2 Cedar Street
Newark, NJ 07102
(201) 733-6437

New Orleans Public Schools' Health Education Program to Prevent the Spread of AIDS
Taylor, S. D.; Glapion, R. E., Jr.
Orleans Parish (New Orleans, Louisiana) School Board
Orleans Parish School Board
Athletics and Physical Education
4100 Touro Street
New Orleans, LA 70116
(504) 942-1714; (504) 483-6444

Project A.R.R.E.S.T.
AIDS Risk Reduction Through Education and Staff Training
Rosica, T. C.
School District of **Philadelphia** (Pennsylvania)
School District of Philadelphia
Office of Categorical Programs
Room 204
21st Street and the Parkway
Philadelphia, PA 19103
(215) 299-7842

San Diego School Health Education AIDS Prevention Project
Fletcher, E. S.
San Diego (California) Unified School District
San Diego Unified School District
Health Services Department
2716 Marcy Avenue
San Diego, CA 92113
(619) 233-8951

School Health Education to Prevent the Spread of AIDS—SAN FRANCISCO TRAINING AND OUTREACH
Lam, Y. M.
City and County of **San Francisco** (California) Unified School District
City and County of San Francisco Unified School District
135 Van Ness Avenue
San Francisco, CA 94102
(415) 565-9613

AIDS Awareness Education Program to Prevent the Spread of the HIV/ AIDS Virus
Iman, J. D.
Seattle (Washington) School District #1
Seattle School District #1
Office of External Funding
814 4th Avenue, North
Seattle, WA 98109
(206) 281-6204

6. Regional AIDS Education and Training Centers (alphabetical by headquarter state)

University of Southern California School of Medicine
1420 San Pablo Street
Los Angeles, **California** 90033
California, Counties of Los Angeles,

Orange, Ventura, Riverside, San Bernadino

University of California, Davis—Department of Family Practice
2221 Stockton Boulevard
Sacramento, **California** 95817
Clark Jones; Dr. Charles Gessert
(209) 252-2851
California, Nevada, Arizona, Hawaii

University of Colorado Health Sciences Center
SEARCH/AHEC Program
4200 E. 9th Avenue, Box A-096
Denver, **Colorado** 80262
Dr. RickiAnn Saylor
(303) 270-5885
North Dakota, South Dakota, Utah, Colorado, New Mexico, Nebraska, Kansas, Wyoming

Emory University School of Medicine
1462 Clifton Road
Atlanta, **Georgia** 30322
Dr. Kathleen R. Miner
(404) 727-7806
Alabama, Georgia, Florida, North Carolina, South Carolina

University of Illinois at Chicago—Department of Medical Social Work
840 S. Wood Street M/C 778
Chicago, **Illinois** 60612
Dr. Nathan L. Linsk
(312) 996-6916
Iowa, Minnesota, Wisconsin, Illinois, Indiana, Missouri

Louisiana State University Medical School
1542 Tulane Avenue
New Orleans, **Louisiana** 70112
Dr. Robert L. Marier
(504) 568-3414
Arkansas, Louisiana, Mississippi

University of Maryland at Baltimore—East Hall
520 West Lombard Street
Baltimore, **Maryland** 21201
Dr. Edward N. Brandt
(301) 328-7004
Maryland, District of Columbia, Virginia, West Virginia, Delaware

Massachusetts Statewide AHEC Program
University of Massachusetts Medical Center
55 Lake Avenue North
Worcester, **Massachusetts** 01655
Michael E. Huppert
(617) 856-3255
Maine, Vermont, New Hampshire, Rhode Island, Massachusetts

New York University School of Education, Health, Nursing and Arts
Division of Nursing
50 W. 4th Street, Room 534
New York, **New York** 10003
Dr. Erline P. McGriff; Dr. Patricia Hurley
(212) 998-5335
New York, New Jersey, Connecticut, Puerto Rico, Virgin Islands

Ohio State University—Department of Family Medicine
B0902 UHC, 456 W. 10th Avenue
Columbus, **Ohio** 43210
Dr. Lawrence L. Gabel
(614) 293-8188
Ohio, Michigan, Kentucky, Tennessee

Knoxville Area Chapter
6921 Middlebrook Pike
P.O. Box 50156
Nashville, **Tennessee** 37950-0156
(615) 584-2999
Coalition for AIDS Education in East Tennessee

The University of Texas at El Paso
College of Nursing and Allied Health
1101 North Campbell
El Paso, **Texas** 79902-0581
(915) 747-5880
Southwest AIDS Committee, Inc.

University of Washington—School of Medicine
SC-64 HSC, E-307
Seattle, **Washington** 98195
Dr. David W. Johnson
(206) 543-6020
Washington, Oregon, Idaho, Alaska

7. Philanthropic Organizations (alphabetical by title)

Otto **Bremer** Foundation
55 E. 5th Street
Suite 700
St. Paul, MN 55101
(612) 227-8036

Supports programs on post-secondary education, human services, health, religions, and community affairs. Giving is limited to area where there are Bremer Bank affiliates: Minnesota, North Dakota, and Wisconsin.

The Cleveland Foundation
1400 Hanna Building
Cleveland, OH 44115
(216) 861-3810

Giving is limited to private tax-exempt and government agencies and programs that serve the greater Cleveland area. Supports programs on civic and cultural affairs, education and economic development, and health and social services.

Columbia Foundation
1090 Sansome Street
San Francisco, CA 94111
(415) 986-5179

Supports general purpose programs that emphasize the arts, environment, human rights and the disadvantaged, community development, neighborhood revitalization and world peace. Giving restricted to Northern California, particularly the San Francisco Bay area.

The Mary A. **Crocker** Trust
233 Post Street
Suite 600
San Francisco, CA 94108
(415) 982-0138

Supports only creative and innovative programs in the San Francisco Bay area.

The B. C. **Gamble** and P. W. Skogmo Foundation
821 Marquette Avenue
Foshay Tower
Suite 500
Minneapolis, MN 55402

Giving is limited to Minneapolis–St. Paul area for programs that deal with disadvantaged youth and their families, and the handicapped. Also, it supports programs in the field of aging, health care, research and education, and higher and secondary education institutions.

Gannett Foundation, Inc.
Lincoln Tower-26th Floor
Rochester, NY 14604
(716) 262-3315

Supports journalism-related programs in communities served by daily newspapers, broadcast stations, outdoor advertising companies, and Gannett Company–owned entities. Program area include: education, charitable, civic, cultural, health and social institutions. Giving is confined to the U.S. and Canada.

Wallace Alexander **Gerbode** Foundation
470 Columbus Avenue
Suite 201
San Francisco, CA 94133
(415) 391-0911

Giving confined to the five San Francisco Bay Area counties and Hawaii. Supports innovative AIDS school education programs.

Hearst Foundation, Inc. and William Randolph Hearst Foundation, Inc.
888 Seventh Avenue
New York, NY 10106
(212) 586-5404

Although the area of giving is broad, these foundations also provide support for public educational and cultural programs.

The James **Irvine** Foundation
One Market Plaza
Steuart Street Tower

Suite 2305
San Francisco, CA 94105
(415) 787-2244
Provides financial support for higher education, health, youth services, community services, and cultural projects. Giving is limited to California.

Ittleson Foundation, Inc.
645 Madison Avenue
New York, NY 10021
(212) 838-5010
Supports research for education, welfare and health programs in the United States.

Marin Community Foundation, CA
1100 Larkspur Landing Circle
Suite 365
Larkspur, CA 94939
(415) 461-3333
Funds nonprofit, charitable, religious, and educational projects, such as AIDS prevention program that targets intravenous drug use. Giving limited to Marin County, CA.

Meadows Foundation, Inc.
2922 Swiss Avenue
Dallas, TX 75204
(214) 826-9431
Although its giving is limited to Texas, this foundation supports arts, social services, health, education, and civic programs.

Eugene and Agnes E. **Meyer** Foundation
1200 15th Street, NW
Suite 500
Washington, DC 20005
(202) 659-2435
Giving is confined to the Washington, DC, area for community development and services, welfare, education and promotion related to AIDS, and pilot projects and school AIDS conferences.

Milwaukee Foundation
161 East Wisconsin Avenue
Suite 5146
Milwaukee, WI 53203
(414) 272-5805
Funds charitable programs that benefit the greater Milwaukee community, particularly to coordinate and expand AIDS volunteer services and education programs.

The Minneapolis Foundation
500 Foshay Tower
821 Marquette Avenue
Minneapolis, MN 55402
(612) 339-7343
Supports AIDS-related programs that provide education and prevention techniques for the Minneapolis–St. Paul area.

The Moody Foundation
704 Moody National Bank Building
Galveston, TX 77550
(409) 763-5333
Supports performing arts organizations and cultural programs that promote health and AIDS education with Texas.

The New York Community Trust
415 Madison Avenue
New York, NY 10017
(212) 758-0100
This is a composite of many charitable funds whose support fund AIDS education and research projects. Priority is given to requests that have significance to the New York City area.

New York Foundation
369 Lexington Avenue
New York, NY 10017
(212) 599-0330
Supports model AIDS programs, AIDS forums, and volunteer services for public education, prevention and social services.

The Pew Memorial Trust
c/o The Glenmede Trust Company
229 South 18th Street
Philadelphia, PA 19103
(215) 875-3200
Giving supports public policy options to AIDS and other human and educational services.

Public Welfare Foundation, Inc.
2600 Virginia Avenue, NW
Room 505
Washington, DC 20037
(202) 965-1800

Supports programs that help reduce the spread of AIDS, education materials, and programs that serve low-income population. Grassroots organizations receive particular consideration.

Rockefeller Brothers Fund
1290 Avenue of the Americas
New York, NY 10104
(212) 397-4800

Funds local, national, and international organizations that emphasize education of high-risk groups, programs for prevention of AIDS, and efforts to develop public policy about AIDS.

The Spencer Foundation
875 North Michigan Avenue
Chicago, IL 60611
(312) 337-7000

Supports organizations that learn and improve AIDS education and community response to children with AIDS.

van Amerigen Foundation, Inc.
509 Madison Avenue
New York, NY 10021
(212) 758-6221

Although giving is limited to urban northeast region of the U.S., funding supports social work and counseling of persons with AIDS.

8. Expert Review Panel (alphabetical by name)

Bruce Anderson, MSW
Deputy Executive Director for Program Operations
Gay Men's Health Crisis
New York, NY
(212) 807-6664

Nancy Nakamura Arnold, JD
Health Policy Consultant
National Minority AIDS Council
Washington, DC
(202) 544-1076

Reverend Carl Bean
Executive Director
Minority AIDS Project/LA
Los Angeles, CA
(213) 936-4949

The Reverend Thaddeus A. Bennett, MDiv
Director
AIDS Ministries Office
Hartford, CT
(203) 233-4481

William A. Bogan
Executive Vice President
National Coalition of Hispanic Health and Human Services Organizations
Washington, DC
(202) 371-2100

Kathleen Bremer
Health Educator
AIDS Education Project
Montefiore Medical Center
Bronx, NY
(212) 920-6741/5431

Doug Conaway, JD
National Coordinator
AIDS Project
American College Health Association
Rockville, MD
(301) 963-1100

Milagros Davilla, MPH
Senior Health Educator
AIDS Program
Los Angeles County Department of Health Services
Los Angeles, CA
(213) 744-3880

Mindy Fullilove, MD
Associate Director
Multicultural Inquiry and Research on AIDS
San Francisco, CA
(415) 822-4030

Aida L. Giachello, MSW
College of Social Work
University of Illinois at Chicago; and the Hispanic Health Alliance
Chicago, IL
(312) 996-0034; (312) 252-6888

Joel Gray, LPN, BSNc
Iowa Center for AIDS/ARC Resources and Education; and National Association of People with AIDS (NAPWA)
Iowa City, IA
(319) 354-1877

Christopher S. Hall
Coordinator
Clearinghouse and Research Development
National AIDS Network
Washington, DC
(202) 347-0390

Trish M. Houtteman
AIDS Education Task Force
UAW-GM Human Resources
Health and Safety Training
Madison Heights, MI
(313) 547-8535

Dianne L. Kerr, MA, MEd
AIDS Education Project Coordinator
American School Health Association
Kent, OH
(216) 678-1601

Iris W. Lee, MPH
Director
Division of AIDS Education
DC Commission of Public Health
Washington, DC
(202) 673-3676

James L. McKittrick, EdD
Director, Medical Services
School of Medicine
University of Alabama
Birmingham, AL
(205) 934-7820

J. Raul Magana, PhD
Supervisor
AIDS Community Project Health Care Agency
County of Orange
Santa Ana, CA
(714) 834-8700

Harvey J. Makadon, MD
Medical Director of Ambulatory Services
Department of Medicine
Beth Israel Hospital
Harvard Medical School; and Executive Director, Boston AIDS Consortium
Boston, MA
(617) 735-3996

Alison Moed, RN, BSN
Head Nurse, 5A
San Francisco General Hospital Medical Center
San Francisco, CA
(415) 821-8153

Patricia Nichols, BSN, MS
Michigan Department of Education
Lansing, MI
(313) 474-8543

Elizabeth Randall-David, RN, PhD
Pediatric Hematology
Program Coordinator
Children's Medical Services
State of Florida/Florida Association of Pediatric Tumor Programs
AIDS Risk Reduction Project
Gainesville, FL
(904) 375-6848

Judith A. Spiegel, MPH
Director of Education and Training
AIDS Project Los Angeles
Los Angeles, CA
(213) 380-2000

Susan Tross, PhD
Clinical Assistant
Psychologist
Psychiatry Service
Memorial Sloan Kettering Cancer Center; and Co-Founder, AIDSFILMS
New York, NY
(212) 207-3276; (212) 629-6288

Armin Weinberg, PhD
Director, Center for Cancer Control Research
Baylor College of Medicine
The Methodist Hospital
Director, Education Division
DeBakey Heart Center
Houston, TX
(713) 799-4614

B. J. Weiss
Associate Director
Health Education and Resources Organization, Inc. (HERO)
Baltimore, MD
(301) 685-1180

James A. Wells, PhD
Senior Policy Analyst
Project HOPE Center for Health Affairs
Chevy Chase, MD
(301) 656-7401

Jim Williams
Director
Health Information Network
National Education Association
Washington, DC
(404) 875-8819; (202) 822-7380

9. Brochure Screening Consultants (alphabetical by name)

Jane L. Delgado, PhD
President
National Coalition of Hispanic Health and Human Services Organizations
Washington, DC
(202) 371-2100

Patricia W. Gillespie, MPH, RPT
Director of Leadership Program American Society of Allied Health Professions
Washington, DC
(202) 857-1150

Jan Mark Orenstein, MD, PhD
Associate Professor
Department of Psychology
George Washington University
Washington, DC
(202) 994-2943

Leonardo Ramon Ortega, MD, MPH
AIDS Coordinator
Office of Latin Affairs
Washington, DC
(202) 328-1238

Sylvia Silver, DA
Associate Professor
Department of Pathology
George Washington University
Washington, DC
(202) 994-2945

Carol Smith, MS
Assistant Professor
Department of Pathology
George Washington University
Washington, DC
(202) 994-2945

Karen E. Spellman
Karen Spellman Enterprises
Washington, DC
(202) 832-4274

Chapter Sixteen

Suggestions for Further Reading

A. ODASUO ALALI

General

Alysou, S. (1988) *You Can Do Something About AIDS.* Boston: The Stop AIDS Project, Inc., 126 pp.

Bayer, R. (1991). *Private Acts, Social Consequences: AIDS and the Politics of Public Health.* New Brunswick, NJ: Rutgers University Press, 302 pp.

Biemiller, L. (1991, December 18). "Campus Health Experts Are Frustrated About Progress on AIDS Education." *The Chronicle of Higher Education,* pp. A-33, A-34.

Center for Population Options (1989, September). *Adolescents, AIDS and HIV: Resources for Educators.* Washington, DC: CPO, 19 pp.

____ (1989, April). *Adolescents, AIDS and HIV: Resources for Educators.* Washington, DC: CPO, 12 pp.

Collins, G. (1987, March 9). "AIDS and TV: What to Tell a Young Child." *New York Times* (Style section).

Curran, W.; Gostin, L.; and Clark, M. (1988). *AIDS: Legal and Regulatory Policy.* Frederick, MD: University Publishing Group, 381 pp.

Delaware State Department of Public Instruction (1989). *Guidelines for a Model HIV/AIDS Infection School District Policy for Students and Employees.* Dover: Delaware State Department of Public Instruction, Author, 7 pp.

De-Vault, C. (1983). *Don't Let It Get Around.* Santa Cruz, CA: Network Publications, 166 pp.

DiGiovanni, C., and Polk, F. (1986). "Adolescents Must Be Taught About Threats of AIDS." *Second Opinion,* pp. 41231–41286.

Freudenberg, N., and Lee, J. (1987). "AIDS Educators' Perceptions of Political Barriers to Effective Health Education: Report on a National Survey." Presented at the annual meeting of the American Public Health Association and sponsored by the American Public Health Association Public Health Education Series.

Fulton, G. B.; Metress, E.; and Price, J. H. (1987, January). "AIDS: Resource Materials for School Personnel." *Journal of School Health,* 57(1):14–18.

Gallup Organization (1985). "Public Awareness of AIDS." Princeton, NJ: Gallup.

Gittlen, M. (1987, November 2). "Credentials of Some Health Teachers Questioned." *Legislative Gazette.*

Hausherr, R. (1989). *Children and the AIDS Virus.* NY: Clarion Books, 48 pp.

Herick, G. M. (1986). "Public Education About AIDS: Is Information Enough?" Presented at the annual convention of the American Psychological Association, New York.

Horan, P. F., and Sherman, R. A. (1988). "School Psychologists and the AIDS Epidemic." *Professional School Psychology,* 3(1):33–49.

Hyde, M. O., and Forsyth, E. H. (1987). *AIDS: What Does It Mean to You?* New York: Walker and Company, 116 pp.

Idaho State Department of Education (1988, September). *School-Based AIDS Policy, Procedures, and Education: A Process Approach.* Boise, ID: Idaho State Department of Education, 255 pp.

Johnson, D. (1987, March). "In Classroom's New Alphabet Lesson, 'A' Is for AIDS." *New York Times.*

Kirp, D. L. (1989). *Learning by Heart: AIDS and School Children in America's Communities.* New Brunswick, NJ: Rutgers University Press, 304 pp.

Koch, J. (1988). *Talking About AIDS: An Understanding.* Rosylyn, NY: Berrent Publications, 64 pp.

Lohrmann, D. K. (1988, October). "AIDS Education at the Local Level: The Pragmatic Issues." *Journal of School Health,* 58(8):330–334.

McCormack, T. P. (1990). *The AIDS Benefits Handbook.* New Haven, CT: Yale University Press, 257 pp.

Macklin, E. A. (1989). *AIDS and Families.* New York: Haworth Press, 284 pp.

Madaras, L. (1988). *Lynda Madaras Talks to Teens: An Essential Guide for Parents, Teachers, and Young People.* New York: New Market Press, 106 pp.

Massachusetts Department of Public Health, AIDS Office (1990). *Comprehensive Guidelines for Adolescent HIV Antibody Counseling and Testing.* Boston: Massachusetts Department of Public Health, 22 pp.

Ministry of Health (1986). *AIDS: Information for Parents and Teachers.* Toronto, Ontario: Ministry of Health.

National Association of State Boards of Education (1989). *Someone at School Has AIDS: A Guide to Developing Policies for Students and School Staff Members Who Are Infected with HIV.* Alexandria, VA: National Association of State Boards of Education, 35 pp.

National Education Association Health Information Network (1989). *Responding to HIV and AIDS.* Morrow, GA: NEA, 34 pp.

Perrow, C., and Guillen, M. F. (1990). *The AIDS Disaster.* New Haven, CT: Yale University Press, 206 pp.

Petrow, S., ed. (1990). *Ending the HIV Epidemic: Community Strategies in Disease Prevention and Health Promotion.* Santa Cruz, CA: Network Publication, 164 pp.

Picchi, J. (1987, April 10). "Campaign Begins to Fight AIDS with Education." *Times Union,* p. B-5.

Price, J. H.; Desmond, S.; and Kukulka, G. (1985). "High School Students' Perceptions and Misperceptions of AIDS." *Journal of School Health,* 55, pp. 107–109.

Public Health Reports (1991, November-December), 106(6).

Puckett, S. B., and Emery, A. R. (1989). *Managing AIDS in the Workplace.* Reading, MA: Addison-Wesley, 191 pp.

Rimmer, S. (1986, February 27). "Volunteers Comfort Lonely AIDS Children." *New York Times,* p. B-1.

Sanchez, J. (1988). "Hispanic AIDS Education in South Texas." *AIDS Information Exchange,* 5(2).

Schachter, V., and Geidt, T. E. (1989). *When an Employee Has AIDS.* New York: Executive Enterprises, Inc., 128 pp.

Schinazi, R. F., and Nahmias, A. J., eds. (1988). *AIDS in Children, Adolescents & Heterosexual Adults: An Interdisciplinary Approach to Prevention.* NY: Elsevier Science Publishing Co.

Shannon, G. W.; Pyle, G. F.; and Bashshur, R. L. (1991). *The Geography of AIDS: Origins and Course of an Epidemic.* New York: The Guilford Press, 192 pp.

Shayne, V. T., and Kaplan, B. J. (1988, December). "AIDS Education for Adolescents." *Youth & Society,* Vol. 20, No. 2, pp. 180–208.

Sieghart, P. (1989). *AIDS and Human Rights: A UK Perspective.* London: British Medical Association Foundation for AIDS, 103 pp.

Sontag, S. (1989). *AIDS and Its Metaphor.* New York: Farrar, Straus & Giroux, 95 pp.

U.S. Conference of Mayors (1987, January). "Local School Districts Active in AIDS Education: 73 City and 25 State Survey Results." *AIDS Information Exchange,* 4.

U.S. Department of Health and Human Services (1989). *Adolescents and School Health Resources: HIV and AIDS. A Cumulation of the AIDS School Health Education Data Base.* Atlanta, GA: U.S. Department of Health and Human Services, 138 pp.

U.S. Department of Justice (1988, July). *Report on Advice to School Superintendents: Planning for the Admission of Students with AIDS and Managing Potentially Adverse Community Reaction.* Philadelphia, PA: U.S. Department of Justice Community Relations Service, 9 pp.

Valdiserri, R. O. (1989). *Preventing AIDS: The Decision of Effective Programs.* New Brunswick, NJ: Rutgers University Press, 304 pp.

Valentich, M., and Gripton, J. (1989, Summer). "Teaching Children About AIDS." *Journal of Sex Education and Therapy,* 15(2):92–102.

Watstein, S. B., and Laurich, R. A. (1991). *AIDS and Women: A Sourcebook.* Phoenix, AZ: Oryx Press, 159 pp.

Weiner, R. C. (1986). *AIDS: Impact on the Schools.* Arlington, VA: Educational Research Group, 274 pp.

Whitmore, G. W. (1988). *Someone Was Here: Profiles in the AIDS Epidemic.* New York: New American Library, 211 pp.

Williams, L. (1988). "AIDS and the Runaway Teenager." In Hines, V. K. (ed.), *1988 American Directory of Programs for Runaways, Homeless Youth and Missing Children,* pp. 4–12. Washington, DC: American Youth Work Center.

Zacarias, F. R. K., ed. (1989). *AIDS: Profile of an Epidemic.* Washington, DC: Pan American Health Organization, 365 pp.

Students

Advocates for Youth (1994). *A Youth Leader's Guide to Building Cultural Competence.* Washington, D.C.: Author, 76 pp.

Blake, J. (1990). *Risky Times: How to Be AIDS Smart and Stay Healthy: A Guide for Teenagers.* New York: Workman Publishing, 158 pp.

Coleman, W. (1988). *Understanding and Preventing AIDS: A Guide for Young People.* Chicago: Children's Press, 123 pp.

Hein, K.; DiGeronimo, F. T.; and the Editors of Consumer Reports Books (1989). *AIDS: Trading Fear for Facts: A Guide for Teens.* Mount Vernon, NY: Consumer Union.

Marsh, C. S. (1988). *First AIDS: Frank Facts for Kids.* Bath, NC: Gallopade Publishing Group, 24 pp.

South Carolina AIDS Education Network, Inc. (1988). *Our Kids Want to Know About AIDS: A Coloring Book.* Columbia: S.C. AIDS Education Network, 10 pp.

Yarber, W. L. (1989). *AIDS: What Young Adults Should Know.* Reston, VA: American Alliance for Health, Physical Education, Recreation, and Dance.

Teacher Preparation/Training

American Medical Students Association (1988). *STATS: Students Teaching AIDS to Students.* Reston, VA: AMSA, 64 pp.

Boston School Committee (1987). *Lesson Plan on AIDS.* Boston: Boston School Committee, 8 pp.

Bradley, B.; Loya, R.; and Van Dellen, L. (1987). *AIDS Prevention Programs for Youth: Information for Teachers/Leaders.* Santa Ana, CA: American Red Cross.

Collins, J. A., and Britton, P. O. (1990). *Training Educators in HIV Prevention, an Inservice Manual.* Santa Cruz, CA: Network Publications, 153 pp.

Colman, W. (1989). *Teacher's Guide for Understanding and Preventing AIDS.* Chicago: Children's Press, 33 pp.

Krim, M. (1987, October). "AIDS: Questions Students Ask." *Scholastic Choices,* 3(2): 29–33, 42.

Meeks, L., and Heit, P. (1988). *AIDS Understanding and Prevention* (Teacher edition). Columbus, OH: Merrill Publishing Co., 26 pp.

Miller, L., and Downer, A. (1988, April). "AIDS: What You and Your Friends Need to Know—A Lesson Plan for Adolescents." *Journal of School Health,* 58(4):137–141.

Montana Office of Public Instruction (1988, September). *AIDS Trainer's Guide: State of Montana.* Helena: Montana Office of Public Instruction, 204 pp.

National Safety Council (1988). *Guide to Teaching About AIDS.* Chicago: NSC, 43 pp.

Planned Parenthood Federation of America (1987). *A Comprehensive Guide to AIDS Information: More Than a Hundred Ways to Teach About AIDS.* New York: PPFA.

Quackenbush, M., and Sargent, P. (1988). *Teaching AIDS: A Resource Guide on Acquired Immune Deficiency Syndrome.* Santa Cruz, CA: Network Publications, 159 pp.

____ and Villarreal, S. (1988). *Does AIDS Hurt?: Educating Young Children About AIDS.* Santa Cruz, CA: Network Publications, 149 pp.

Sroka, S. R. (1989). *Educator's Guide to AIDS and Other STD's.* Lakewood, OH: Health Education Consultants, 76 pp.

Tatum, M. L. (1988, Fall). "The AIDS Challenge: Controversial Issues in the Classroom." *Family Life Educator,* 7(1):15–19.

Waples, R. A. (1987, December). "AIDS and the Science Teacher." *Hoosier Science Teacher,* 13(2):58–62.

White, D. M., and Matthews, S. (1988, October). "AIDS and the Immune System: Teaching Techniques." *Journal of School Health,* 58(8):339–340.

Yarber, W. L. (1993). *STDs and HIV: A Guide for Today's Young Adults. Instructor's Guide.* Reston, VA: American Alliance for Health, Physical Education, Recreation and Dance, 98 pp.

Curriculum Development

Brick, P. (1989). *Teaching Safer Sex.* Hackensack, NJ: Planned Parenthood of Bergen County, 92 pp.

Brown, L. K., and Fritz, G. K. (1988, July). "AIDS Education in the Schools: A Literature Review as a Guide for Curriculum Planning." *Clinical Pediatrics,* 27(7):311–316.

Carrera, J. W. (1989). *Immigrant Students: Their Legal Right to Access to Public Schools.* Boston: National Coalition of Advocates for Students, 63 pp.

Center for Population Options (1988). *Life Planning Education: A Youth Development Program.* Washington, DC: CPO, 372 pp.

Centers for Disease Control (1988, January 29). "Guidelines for Effective School Health Education to Prevent the Spread of AIDS." *Morbidity and Mortality Weekly Report,* 37(2):14 pp.

Connecticut Department of Education (1988, November). *Acquired Immunodeficiency Syndrome (AIDS): Primary and Elementary Levels.* Hartford, CT: Connecticut Department of Education, 29 pp.

Dickman, I. R. (1982). *Winning the Battle for Sex Education.* New York: SIECUS, 58 pp.

Dodge, S. (1991, December 18). "A Course on AIDS and Society Covers Science, History, Sociology, and Politics of the Disease." *The Chronicle of Higher Education,* pp. A-33, A-34.

Dorman, S. M.; Small, P. A.; and Lee, D. D. (1989, September). "Cooperative Learning Techniques for AIDS Education. *Journal of School Health,* 59(9):408–409.

Educational Development Center, Inc. (1989). *Integrating AIDS into Teenage Health Teaching Modules.* Newton, MA: EDC, 122 pp.

Florida Department of Education (1988). *AIDS Education and Prevention.* Tallahassee: Florida Department of Education, 484 pp.

Gelber, S. (1988, January-February). "Developing an AIDS Program in a Juvenile Detention Center." *Children Today,* 17(1):6–9.

Hylton, J. (1992). *SAFE: Stopping AIDS through Functional Education.* Portland, OR: Child Development and Rehabilitation Center, 200 pp.

Kansas State Department of Education (1988). *Human Sexuality and AIDS Education Guidelines. Part 1—Program Development and Resource Selection.* Topeka: Kansas State Department of Education, 31 pp.

____ (1988). *Human Sexuality and AIDS Education Guidelines. Part 2—Curriculum and Staff Development.* Topeka: Kansas State Department of Education, 52 pp.

Kerr, D. L. (1989, November). "New Resources Supplement HIV Education Programs for Adolescents." *Journal of School Health,* 59(9):408–409.

National Coalition of Advocates for Students (1990, May). *On the Road to Healthy Living: A Bilingual Curriculum on AIDS and HIV Prevention for Migrant Students (Grades 6–12).* Boston: NCAS, 345 pp.

____ (1988). *Steps to Help Your School Set Up an AIDS Education Program.* Boston: NCAS, 19 pp. (also available in Haitian Kreyol and Spanish).

Oklahoma State Department of Education (1987). *Acquired Immune Deficiency Syndrome (AIDS) Prevention Education: Curriculum Guide for Teachers.* Oklahoma City: Oklahoma State Department of Education, 49 pp.

Pennsylvania Association for Supervision and Curriculum Development (1987). *Guidelines for Integrating AIDS Education into the Health Education Program.* McMurray: Pennsylvania Association for Supervision and Curriculum Development, 32 pp.

Post, J., and McPherson, C. (1988, August-September). "AIDS: The Truth About Myths." *Health Education Research: Theory and Practice,* 3(1):105–112.

Quackenbush, M.; Nelson, M.; and Clark, K., eds. (1988). *AIDS Challenge: Prevention Education for Young People.* Santa Cruz, CA: Network Publications, 526 pp.

Stangle, J. (1991). *Special Education: Secondary F.L.A.S.H. (Family Life and Sexual Health): A Curriculum for 5th through 10th Grades.* Seattle, WA: Seattle-King County Department of Public Health, 301 pp.

Yarber, W. L. (1987). *AIDS Education: Curriculum and Health Policy.* Bloomington, IN: Phi Delta Kappa Educational Foundation, 58 pp.

About the Contributors

A. Odasuo Alali, the editor, is a recipient of the American Library Association Publishing Committee's Whitney-Carnegie Award (1994). Alali earned his Ph.D. in mass communication from Howard University (1985); he is currently an associate professor of communications at California State University, Bakersfield. He is an active scholar and is the author or co-editor of such books as *Terrorism and the News Media* (McFarland, 1994), *Mass Media Sex and Adolescent Values* (McFarland, 1991), and *Media Coverage of Terrorism: Methods of Diffusion* (Sage, 1991). His articles have appeared in such scholarly journals as *Omega, Psychological Reports, Education, College Student Journal, A Current Bibliography on African Affairs, COMBRAOD* (London) and the *Journal of Black Studies.*

Danny J. Ballard is an associate professor of health education in the Department of Health and Kinesiology at Texas A&M University, College Station. Previously, she was on the faculty at Idaho State University. Ballard, who holds professional membership and elected offices in numerous health-related organizations, has contributed articles to books and has published numerous articles in refereed journals. She is under contract to write a women's health textbook. She has served as keynote speaker at national, regional and state conventions.

Benjamin W. Brucker is a professor of education at Eastern Washington University at Cheney, Washington. His teaching experience includes work at the elementary and secondary levels. He has written numerous articles for professional journals and has made many presentations at major conferences. Brucker earned his B.A. from Gonzaga University in Spokane, Washington, his M.Ed. from Eastern Washington University, and his Ed.D. from Arizona State University in Tempe, Arizona.

Gary Byrd is associate professor of communication at California State University, Bakersfield. He holds a Ph.D. in instructional technology from the University of Oklahoma, where he also obtained a master of science degree in Education. His professional accomplishments in the area include work in language skills development and interactive media. He has numerous audiovisual productions and research to his credit.

Fidelis Ejianreh is a medical student at the University of Medicine & Dentistry of New Jersey. He was a biology teacher at Hollywood High School, Hollywood, California, from 1986 to 1994. Prior to joining the Hollywood High School faculty in 1986, Ejianreh taught biology and chemistry in the Cleveland City Schools between 1983 and 1986. Ejianreh has a bachelor's degree from Alabama A&M University (1980) and a master's degree in secondary education from California State University at Los Angeles (1989).

Larry D. Farrell has a B.S. (1964) and an M.S. (1966) in microbiology from the University of Oklahoma. His Ph.D. (1972) in bacteriology is from the University of California, Los Angeles. From 1970 to 1972 he served as a postdoctoral fellow and instructor at the University of Illinois College of Medicine. Currently he is a professor of microbiology in the Department of Biological Sciences at Idaho State University, Pocatello. His research interests include bacterial viruses of *Sphaerotilus natans* (a sheathed bacterium) and HIV/AIDS education. He is widely published, examples of his work having appeared in *Antimicrobial Agents and Chemotherapy, The Canadian Journal of Microbiology, Education,* and *The Clearinghouse.*

James T. Girvan is a professor and chair of the Department of Health and Nutrition Sciences at Idaho State University. He received his Ph.D. in health education from the University of Oregon in 1986. Prior to that, he taught both general and advanced placement chemistry in high school in Tacoma, Washington, for 13 years. Girvan has published 20 articles on school health curriculum, school health methods, HIV/AIDS, health program evaluation, and behavior change strategies. In addition, he has written a junior high school curriculum on HIV/AIDS and has given over 200 comprehensive in-service presentations to various school and community groups on HIV/AIDS and other health topics. His research interests include disease prevention strategies, comprehensive school health programs, health program planning and evaluation, and strategies for changing or adopting positive health behaviors.

Wayne H. Hall received his Ph.D. in mathematics and educational psychology from George Peabody College for Teachers in 1970 and has been actively involved in teacher education for his entire career. For the past 24 years he has been a member of the mathematics and education faculties. At this writing he is the director of the Bureau of Educational Research in the Department of Education at Eastern Washington University. His primary interest is in program evaluation and the teaching of mathematics, with numerous articles related to the teaching of mathematics.

Doris Helge is a prominent author in the areas of rural education, rural special education, children at risk, and HIV/AIDS education. She has produced books and journals in these areas. In addition, she has conducted national research and other projects concerning the above topics. She is a frequent keynote speaker at national and regional conferences in her fields. She is a private consultant with Perpetual Resources in Ferndale, Washington.

Daryl L. Hitchcock is now completing his Ph.D. in clinical psychology at the California School of Professional Psychology, Fresno, CA. While he was pursuing his undergraduate degree in psychology at California State University, Bakersfield, he developed a specialized interest in social issues related to prejudice, heterosexism, feminism, and deafness. He was a founding officer of the CSUB Psychology Club, founding president of the CSUB Chapter of Psi Chi national Honor Society for Psychology, and an active member of the CSUB Gay and Lesbian Academic Union.

B. A. Jinadu, M.D., M.P.H., is a board certified pediatrician, and is currently the director of public health services and health officer for the County of Kern, California.

M. David Miller is with the University of Florida, Gainesville. A well-known researcher in the field, Miller has distinguished himself in research about AIDS, particularly as it relates to education and public policy. His research findings have been published in refereed journals such as *AIDS Education and Prevention.*

National Coalition of Advocates for Students (NCAS) is a national network of 23 experienced child advocacy organizations that work to improve access to quality education for all children, particularly those who are members of racial or linguistic minorities, recently immigrated, and or physically challenged. The NCAS provides resources for schools, parents, and advocates.

Beth M. Rienzi obtained her Ph.D. in clinical psychology from the California School of Professional Psychology–Fresno in 1983. She has been a licensed psychologist in the state of California since 1985 and started her academic career in 1988 at California State University, Bakersfield, where she completed her undergraduate degree in psychology and is now an associate professor. Her teaching responsibilities include graduate level psychology of human sexuality for the Marriage, Family, Child Counselor program. Her research interests include gay and lesbian issues, deafness, substance abuse, and forensic psychology.

Gordon Thornton is a faculty member in the College of Education at the University of Florida, Gainesville. Thorton's research has been applied by experts in death education and counseling as well as scholars in the field. Some of his research can be found in *AIDS Education and Prevention,* a leading international journal on AIDS education and prevention.

Wemme E. Walls is the director of academic support services at the Citadel in Charleston, South Carolina, and previously served as the director of the Institute for the Study of Exceptionalities, College of Education, Virginia Polytechnic Institute and State University. Walls has prevented policy papers at state and national conferences and seminars on educational placement issues for students with HIV. At this writing, she is researching policy issues for students with disabilities in post-secondary programs.

Hannelore Wass is on the faculty at the University of Florida, Gainesville, and is the founding editor of the journal *Death Studies.* She is widely published, and her research has received both national and international recognition.

David M. White is an associate professor of health education at East Carolina University, Greenville, North Carolina. White has published numerous articles on health education and AIDS in the past few years. He is a distinguished scholar whose research has received critical acclaim.

The **Working Group** that developed "Guidelines" comprised representatives from the American Association for Counseling and Development; American Federation of Teachers; American Psychological Association; American School Health Association; National Association of School Nurses; National Association of School Psychologists; National Association of Social Workers, Education Commission; National Association of State School Nurse Consultants; and National Coalition of Advocates for Students. The group's contribution to this book is endorsed by the Midwest School Social Work Council; National Council of State Consultants for School Social Work Services; and National Education Association Health Information Network.

Index

Abstinence 15, 40, 53, 56, 137; teaching about 80
Adolescents: misconception about AIDS 20; risk of HIV infection 72
AFRAIDS (Acute fear relating to AIDS) 31, 75, 145
AIDS: across rural America 51, 130; belief systems, stereotypical 51; cases worldwide, 11; curriculum in rural schools 71–75; definitions 138; discrimination against people with 3; education about 4; litigation on 103; prevention programs 73; preventive measures 15, 56, 59–60; right of a student with 3; school attendance policy for children with 3; and school health programs 53; social fear of 29; spread of 3; student misconceptions about 48; teacher attitudes toward 85–95; treatment of persons with 12
AIDS education: advisory committee and 74; barriers to 72–73; community-based resources and 126–129; criteria for evaluating 130–143; curricula 15; culture and 17–18; effectiveness of 15; elementary grades and 78; goals of 52; high school, at a typical urban 40–50; in-service trainings 75; integrating community-based resources into 124–129; and language 53; mandate 26, 63; materials 48; obstacle to 125; opposition to 48; parents and 48; prevalence of 24; primary goals of 14; public schools 14, 20–28; questionnaire 22; resources 47; rural schools 51–70; rural school administrators and 72; sample letter to parents 17; and sex education 21; teacher preparation and material selection 16–17
AIDS testing: mandatory 85
Alali, A. O. 7, 11, 29, 124, 144, 154, 168, 189
Alan Guttmacher Institute 21
Albert, E. 31
Allensworth, D. 84
Ambrosio, A. L. 29
American Academy of Pediatrics 20, 104; Committee on School Health 20
American Association of Colleges in Teacher Education (AACTE) 78–79
American Association of School Administrators 20
American Council on Rural Special Education 65
American Federation of Teachers 102
American Red Cross 65, 80–82
Anti-discrimination law 105
Apuzzo, V. 32
Ashe, Arthur 30, 104
Associated Press 85
Audiovisual media: goals for 156–157; guidelines for selecting 146–153; importance of 145–146; ordering information 165–167; recommended 157–164; selected 154–164; selecting and evaluating 144–153

Baldwin, D. C. 32
Ballard, D. J. 77–78

Baltimore: clinics and treatment of STDs 12; inner-city teenage girls 12
Beck, K. H. 146, 155
Bouton, R. A. 29, 31, 34–35
Brucker, B. W. 85
Buchanan, Patrick 32
Byrd, G. 154

Campeau, P. L. 143, 146, 154
Center for Health Promotion and Education 21
Center for Population Options (CPO) 14, 156–157; Teens for AIDS Prevention (TAP) 128
Centers for Disease Control (CDC) 11, 21, 64, 78, 80, 82, 85–86, 100–102, 104, 107–108, 114, 146; adolescent School Health 157; national guidelines 101
Child: sex abuse and HIV infection 55; sexual abuse prevention and treatment programs 61
Coalition of National Health Education Organizations, the 20
Cohn, Roy 30
Community-based: advocacy 128; efforts 61; organizations (CBOs) 126; peer education, 127; resources 126–129; resources and school health educators 126; support programs 128
Condom 12, 53; campaigns 45; education 60; program 47; use 137
Council of Exceptional Children 102
Counseling programs 54
Curriculum guidelines 81–82

de Mauro, D. 15
District of Columbia 33
Dropout prevention programs 54

Eastern Washington University 85–86
Education Research Group 56
Ejianreh, F. 4, 40

Family Education Rights and Privacy Act (FERPA) 102
Farrell, L. D. 5, 71
Fear of AIDS: irrational 34; as a media construct 30–31; physical anxiety and 34–35; rational 34; and the school system 36–37; social 34
Ficarrotto, T. J. 33
Forrest, J. D. 16, 25–26, 40, 125

Gallaher, P. E. 29, 31
Garlinghouse, P. A. 29, 31
Gay: bashing 37; men 1; students 37, 121; youth and special needs 141
Gayle, J. 77
Girvan, J. T. 5, 71–72
Glascoff, M. 78
Good, L. R. 34
Gotlieb, M. 1

Haaga, D. 33
Hall, W. H. 85
Harney, D. M. 12
Health educators: survey of 26
Healthy People 2000: National Health Promotion and Disease Promotion Objectives 77
Helge, D. 4, 51
Helms, Jesse 31
Hemophiliacs 1; with AIDS 13
Hepatitis B virus (HBV) 102
Herpes simplex virus (HSV) 102
HIV: curriculum in rural schools 71–75; definition of 138; litigation and legislation 103; privacy of those infected with 4; test counseling and support 117–118; transmission of 138; youth and 112
HIV education: advisory committee and 74–75; age-appropriate 77; appropriate approaches to 135–138; barriers to 72–73; cases in children 100; and community-based solutions 65–66; and extended families 65; high school, at a typical urban 40–50; in-service trainings 75; and language 53; mandated 130; and migrant student 66–67; parental and community involvement 142–143; placement and availability of 53; placement of students with 99–108; prevention programs 73; as a public school issue 100–102; rural school administrators and 72; rural schools 51–70; and school health pro-

gram, 53; and self-esteem education 64; social issues and 137
HIV infected: policy regarding the attendance of 54
HIV infection: avoiding 140; spectrum of 139; testing for 139
Hippocrates 151
Hitchcock, D. L. 29
Homophobia: and heterosexism 33; and IVDU; fear of AIDS and 29–34
Homosexuality: AIDS and 30; denial of existence of 37
House Select Committee on Children, Youth and Families 125
Howe, A. C. 156
Hudson, Rock 30, 32
Hughes, T. 2
Human T Lymphocyte Virus III (HTLV III) 1

Intravenous drug users (IVDU) 1, 30, 51; and sexuality activity 57

Jinadu, B. A. 2
Johnson, Earvin "Magic" 12, 104
Jorgansen, S. 57

Kann, L. 72
Kaplan, B. J. 124
Kerr, D. 77
Koch, Ed 32
Koop, C. Everett 20, 25–26
Kreps, G. 144, 154

L. Harris and Associates 56
Lazes, P. M. 152
Leal, T. 29, 31
Lennon, R. 29
Lesbian: students 121; youth and special needs 141
Liberace 30
Los Angeles Unified School District 48
Luty, E. T. 73

McDevitt, T. M. 29, 35
Martinez v. School Board 106
Mass media: AIDS and 30–31, 85, 104–105; and sexual socialization of the youth 57, 61
Men's Reproductive Center 57
Miller, M. D. 20

Nardi, P. 30
National AIDS Information Clearinghouse 126
National Association of State Boards of Education 21
National Coalition of Advocates for Students 6, 130
National Education Association 102
National Rural and Small Schools Consortium 63
National School Boards Association 14
National Urban League 64
New England Journal of Medicine 12
New York City Board of Education 13
New York Post 32
New York Times 32
Northeastern University 56
Nugent, G. C. 156

Obituaries 30–31

Painter, K. 55
Parents: communication with 58
Parker, C. C. 34
Paulk, J. 57–58
Pediatric AIDS 115–116
Political conservatives: Homophobia and AIDS 31
Public Health Service 21
Public schools: AIDS in 12

Ray v. School District of DeSoto County 13
Red Cross *see* American Red Cross
Rehabilitation Act of 1973 102, 107
Religion: homophobia and AIDS 32
Report of the Surgeon General's Workshop on Children with HIV Infection and Their Families 104
Resources directory 168–188; brochure screening consultants 188; expert review panel 186–188; local school health programs 181–182; national 169–170;

national school health programs 174–175; philanthropic organizations 183–186; regional AIDS education and training centers 182–183; state school health programs 175–180; state public health departments 170–173
Rienzi, B. M. 29
Risk prevention programs 54
Roper, W. L. 12
Rosenstein, L. D. 29, 31

Safer sex 53
Salzman, S. A. 72
Sawyer, R. G. 153, 155
School-based: clinics 64, 124; programs 14
School Board of Nassau County v. Arline 13, 103, 105
School-community partnerships 68
Schumaker, A. M. 105
Self-esteem education 64
Sex: and elementary schools 63; and peer pressure 62
Sex Information and Education Council of the United States (SIECUS) 15
Sexuality education 61–62: conservative schools and 55; curricula 41; problems with existing 57–58; and rural educators 67; success factors in teen 58–60
Sexual orientation: confusion regarding HIV/AIDS and 29–39; diversity of 36
Sexually transmitted diseases (STDs) 12, 55, 116, 138
Shalwitz, J. 55
Shayne, V. T. 124
Sheehan, E. P. 29
Silverman, J. 16, 25–26, 40, 125
Silverman, M. 71
Snyder, D. 152
Stein, D. 149
Student support services: barriers to delivery of 113–114; checklist for evaluating HIV 121–122; components of an HIV 114–121; guidelines for HIV and AIDS 110–122; need for HIV-related 113; policymaking and 119–120; referral and coordination of 118–119; staff training and 120–121
Students: immigrant 127; policy on school attendance of HIV-infected 111; sexually active 12
Suggestions for further readings 189–193
Suicide prevention programs 53
Surgeon General's Report on AIDS 26
Suter, E. 148

Teachers: professional preparation of preservice elementary 77–84; specialized training of 141–142; training programs and AIDS curriculum 85
Teens: and IVDU 55; pregnancy and birth control 64; primary causes of HIV infection amongst 60; and sex 60; and STDs 55
Thomas, R. 13
Thomas v. Atascadero 102
Thornton, G. 20

U.S. Department of Education 21
U.S. Department of Health and Human Services 21
University of California at Los Angeles 1

Vasu, E. S. 156
VFW 65

Waddell, W. H. 148
Walls, M. 5, 13, 99
Wass, H. 20
White, D. M. 77–78
White, Ryan 2, 12, 30, 103
White v. Western School Corp. 103
Will, G. F. 30
Working Group 110
World Health Organization 11
Worth, D. 17

YMCA 63
Young, R. K. 29, 31
YWCA 63